Zhamshid Arslonovich Norchaev

COMPREHENSIVE TREATMENT OF DIABETIC FOOT SYNDROME

Zhamshid Arslonovich Norchaev

COMPREHENSIVE TREATMENT OF DIABETIC FOOT SYNDROME

ScienciaScripts

Cover image: www.ingimage.com

This book is a translation from the original published under ISBN 978-3-659-82253-7.

Publisher:
Sciencia Scripts
is a trademark of
Dodo Books Indian Ocean Ltd. and OmniScriptum S.R.L publishing group

120 High Road, East Finchley, London, N2 9ED, United Kingdom
Str. Armeneasca 28/1, office 1, Chisinau MD-2012, Republic of Moldova, Europe
Managing Directors: Ieva Konstantinova, Victoria Ursu
info@omniscriptum.com

Printed at: see last page
ISBN: 978-620-8-36633-9

JAMSHID ARSLONOVICH NORCHAEV

COMPREHENSIVE TREATMENT OF DIABETIC FOOT SYNDROME

TABLE OF CONTENTS

INTRODUCTION 3

PURULENT-NECROTIC COMPLICATIONS OF THE LOWER LIMBS IN DIABETES MELLITUS 5

RESULTS OF COMPLEX TREATMENT OF DIABETIC FOOT SYNDROME 16

COMPARATIVE ANALYSIS OF THE EFFECTIVENESS OF THE PROPOSED TREATMENT METHODS AND DEVELOPMENT OF A ALGORITHM OF THERAPEUTIC AND DIAGNOSTIC MEASURES FOR SDS 52

WHY E 59

REFERENCE LIST 70

INTRODUCTION

The problem of diabetes mellitus (DM) remains one of the most pressing medical and social problems due to its widespread prevalence, tendency to increase in frequency, severity of numerous complications that are difficult to treat [66, 103]. According to WHO data, there are 170 million people suffering from DM in the world [126]. According to WHO forecasts, the total number of patients with diabetes, which was 120 million in 1996, will increase by 1996. 120 million people, will increase to 250 million by 2025 [122]. [122]. Diabetic foot syndrome (DFS) is one of the complications of diabetes mellitus that most often leads to disability and reduced quality of life, occurring in 15% of patients [138]. In the USA, of the 16 million patients with diabetes, 1.5 million have ulcerative foot disease [174], accounting for 20% of all surgical hospitalisations and 50% of all non-traumatic amputations [154]. One in two patients with diabetes mellitus undergoes surgery, with one in four for a purulent-necrotic complication in the lower limbs [119]. Lower limb amputations in patients in this group are performed 15 times more often than in the rest of the population [103]. From 50 to 70% of the total number of all lower limb amputations is accounted for by patients with DM [51]. According to Muller J.S. (2002) and Benotmane A. (2001), the amputation rate in patients with DM is 17.4-23%, and mortality reaches 9.1%. Annually in the world the number of high amputations of lower limbs in patients with DM exceeds 200 000 [251]. Within 3 years after amputation 35% patients die [129]. The results of studies have shown the need to manage patients taking into account the clinical forms of SDS, the depth and spread of purulent necrotic process. Various methods of surgical treatment of neuropathic and ischaemic forms of SDS have been proposed, indications and contraindications for their performance have been developed [46, 95]. It is known that neuropathy, ischaemia and infection play a major role in the development of purulent-necrotic processes in the lower extremities. In recent years, studies have been conducted to diagnose and treat bone and joint changes in SDS, to identify the place of osteoarthropathy in the development of purulent necrotic complications of the lower limbs in SDS. The frequency of DOAP varies from 1 to 55%. Such inconsistency of data is associated with differences in the methods of examination and different criteria for diagnosing osteoarthropathy [33, 79, 113]. Therapeutic and diagnostic measures aimed at early detection and treatment of the osteoarthropathic form of SDS are not sufficiently developed. The proposed methods of treatment due to ineffectiveness have not been widely used. There are no specific indications and contraindications for conservative and surgical treatment of diabetic osteoarthropathy. The significance of bone changes in the development of SDS and its complications remains controversial. Local therapy of purulent-necrotic processes in the lower extremities in DM with proteolytic enzymes occupies one of the main places in the in the arsenal of therapeutic measures for SDS. Preparations of enzymes isolated from microbial and animal material are widely recognised [3, 33, 34], but preparations of proteolytic enzymes isolated from plants are no less promising [57, 97]. The disadvantage of proteolytic enzymes is their rapid inactivation under the influence of denaturing agents and pH fluctuations. Therefore, proteolytic enzymes have certain requirements: to be resistant, stable to the influence of denaturing agents and to keep high activity at different parameters of ph of purulent-necrotic process. In vivo, a biocatalyst is found among a huge set of other macromolecules, so the choice of enzyme mixture is of particular interest [84]. Analysis of the information of recent years indicates the possibility and prospectivity of using a complex of proteolytic enzymes of the latex of Carica papaya fruits, which includes cucumazyme.Purulent-necrotic processes in the lower extremities in SDS are accompanied by pronounced functional-organic disorders of vital organs and systems. These conditions require the development of such methods of complex therapy, which should be highly effective, accessible, easy to use and have an impact on all pathogenetic links of SDS. In recent years, physical methods of treatment are widely used in the complex of therapeutic measures of purulent-inflammatory diseases. There are reports on the use of autotransfusion of ultraviolet irradiated blood and ultrasound cavitation in the treatment of purulent wounds [54, 77, 109, 153]. However, in the literature, the results of the effectiveness of these methods in the treatment of SDS remain controversial. Classification of purulent-necrotic lesions of the lower extremities in SDS should reflect the etiopathogenesis of the lesion, allow to determine the treatment tactics, have prognostic significance, and be easy to use [8, 95]. In turn, each form of SDS requires detailing the nature, depth, and extent of the lesion with registration of the developing purulent-necrotic complications. However, the proposed classifications of SDS do not fully meet these requirements.Recently in the literature there have appeared works that present the results of analyses of the main causes of low efficiency of care for patients with SDS [90]. The main therapeutic and diagnostic errors are considered to be the lack of a differentiated approach to clinical forms of SDS and incorrect assessment of the severity of SDS without taking into account physical, laboratory and instrumental data. It is necessary to develop an algorithm of therapeutic and diagnostic measures in SDS, which allows timely identification of clinical forms and stages of SDS and to develop gentle methods of complex treatment of destructive forms of diabetic foot, aimed at preserving the support function of the foot [43].

PURULENT-NECROTIC COMPLICATIONS OF THE LOWER LIMBS IN DIABETES MELLITUS

Currently, the number of DM patients worldwide exceeds 170 million [22]. The dynamics of the increasing incidence of foot involvement show that 15% of the more than 170 million patients with DM worldwide have or will have anatomical or pathological changes in the lower extremities with a wide range of foot problems [139,140]. A report by a WHO study group identified "diabetic foot" as a distinct disease [22,150].

Diabetic foot syndrome (DFS) is a pathological condition of the feet of a DM patient, which occurs against the background of peripheral nerve, vascular, skin and soft tissue, bone and joint lesions and creates conditions for the formation of acute and chronic ulcers, bone and joint lesions and purulent-necrotic processes [38]. Diabetic gangrene, which develops as a consequence of untimely diagnosed or inadequately treated SDS, ranks first among the causes of non-traumatic amputations [14]. Annually in the world the number of high amputations of lower limbs in patients with DM exceeds 200000, 11000 of them in Russia [15,74]. Taking into account the prevalence of patients with DM, high frequency of SDS in 1989 the governments of European countries, USA, some Asian countries signed the St. Vincent Declaration on the basis of which a programme on prevention and treatment of DM was developed, according to which in many countries of the world specialised centres for service of patients with purulent-necrotic complications in the lower extremities were created.

The pathogenesis of SDS is extremely complex and, taking into account age-related changes, includes angio, osteo and neuropathy typical of diabetes [4,20,49,113], against which severe purulent-necrotic processes characterised by a specific composition of microflora develop [162,192].The main factors in the development of diabetic foot ulcer are neuropathy and ischaemia [124].

The formation of neuropathy is based on a variety of pathogenetic mechanisms, which are essentially divided into two main categories - metabolic and vascular [38]. The metabolic category includes activation of the polyol pathway of glucose metabolism, oxidative stress, and impaired growth factor formation [162]. The vascular category includes microvascular nerve insufficiency (vaza nervorum) [174]. Disturbances of metabolism and blood flow in the nerve fibre are interrelated at different stages of the pathogenesis of diabetic neuropathy. Chronic hyperglycaemia plays a key role in the pathogenesis of neuropathy. DCCT (Diabetes Control and Complication Trial) studies proved that it is hyperglycaemia that is responsible for the development of diabetic neuropathy [145]. Clinically, neuropathy is manifested by the progressive development of pain and temperature anaesthesia, as well as decreased tactile, vibratory and proprioceptive sensitivity [183]. With progressive loss of weakness of the muscles of the foot develops. Dysfunction of flexor and extensor muscles leads to the formation of typical neuropathic deformities. In addition, neuropathy leads to a decrease in capillary tone, paralytic dilation of shunts, pathological discharge of blood from arteries into veins and contributes to the formation of a destructive process of soft tissues of the foot with preserved main blood flow. Diabetic neuropathy is the cause of SDS development in 70% of cases [28].

Among the vascular lesions of the lower limbs in diabetes, 3 types can be distinguished: lesions of large arterial trunks; lesions of medium and small diameter arteries; and microvascular lesions characterised by thickening of the basement membrane of arterioles and capillaries, which is a diabetes-specific vascular lesion. Histological studies of the vascular system in DM patients and non-diabetic individuals show the same changes [118]. However, diabetic macroangiopathy and obliterative atherosclerosis have fundamental differences. DM patients are characterised by rapid development of changes, younger age, approximately equal incidence in men and women, and asymptomatic course (associated with the presence of neuropathy) [14]. Lower limb ischaemia in DM is detected in 3-7% [38,125].

Despite such conflicting data on the incidence of bone damage in DM, still most clinicians consider diabetic osteoarthropathy as a specific manifestation of bone damage in insulin deficiency [60].

To assess the purulent-necrotic process, radiography of the foot in two projections, radioisotope examination of the foot, computed tomography of the foot; bacteriological, immunological, morphological studies are performed [103]. In the assessment of neurological status, various types of sensitivity are determined: vibration (graduated tuning fork, biotensiometer), tactile (set of monofilaments), temperature (thermal device - Thim-term), pain (using a blunt needle, neurological pen - Neuropen, toothed wheel - Pin-wheel) [4,37]. Pupyshev M.L. (2001) studied the morphology of the tarsal canal and the tibial nerve passing in it in 157 patients with SDS. In 68 patients with neuropathy, the difference in the diameter of the tibial nerve before entering the tarsal canal (0.51±0.04 cm) and along its length (0.77±0.28 cm) was found.

When assessing regional blood flow and microcirculation, investigations should be aimed at diagnosing microangiopathy and macroangiopathy. The simplest way is to determine the pulsation on the main arteries of the lower limb. Angiographic studies are performed to detect the level of occlusion [46]. But, currently, ultrasound Doppler ultrasonography with determination of ankle-shoulder index is considered the most informative and more accessible

[25,62,137]. Additional methods are methods of X-ray contrast angiography with obligatory contrast of the distal arterial channel with pharmacological test; determination of transcutaneous oxygen tension at the first interfinger interval [163], laser Doppler fluorometry (Transonic) [63,179].

Recently, ultrasound echosteometry has been successfully used in the diagnosis of DOAP, the informativity of which, according to some authors, reaches up to 95% [25,67]. Bone biopsy is the "gold standard" in the diagnosis of DOAP [114].

For an objective assessment of the nature of lesions and an accessible comparison of treatment efficacy, the same approach is required, which is provided by the accepted classifications [7]. The current classifications of SDS can be divided into 3 groups [91,118,213]:

1. By etiological and pathogenetic principle;
2. By clinical and morphological principle;
3. Combined classifications.

The WHO (1987) classification is based on etiopathogenetic aspects, where 3 forms of diabetic foot are distinguished:

1. Neuropathic foot is up to 70% [38].
2. Ischaemic foot is 3-7% [46,49].
3. Neuroischaemic foot is 25-30%.

The classification of Wagner S. is widely spread abroad. [251], which takes into account clinical forms and the depth of the necrotic process, which includes 5 stages:

-0 stage - without purulent-necrotic changes of the foot;
-I-II stage - superficial trophic changes and perforating ulcers;
-III stage - deep damage - abscess, phlegmon, necrosis, osteomyelitis;
-IV stage - gangrene of the toes;
-V stage - widespread gangrene of the foot.

The treatment of purulent necrotic lesions of the lower limbs in patients with DM remains a challenge. The combination of DM and surgical infection forms a vicious circle in which the infection negatively affects metabolic processes, exacerbating insulin deficiency and increasing acidosis, and metabolic and microcirculatory disorders worsen the course of reparative processes in the lesion [39]. The combination of these diseases worsens the prognosis, as there is a danger of spreading infection, on the one hand, and a continuous increase in ketoacidosis up to the development of diabetic coma and endotoxemia, on the other [29,30,31,48]. Treatment of purulent-necrotic lesions of the lower extremities is carried out taking into account the type of infection [192], the state of blood flow, phase and localisation of the inflammatory process, peculiarities of general and local manifestations due to the properties of pathogens and immunological reactivity of the patient's organism [81,189]. In this regard, treatment is mainly complex and includes the use of surgical and conservative methods and means aimed at normalisation of carbohydrate, protein and electrolyte metabolism, acid-base balance, elimination of purulent focus, impact on microflora, detoxification, restoration of disturbed functions of vital organs and stimulation of natural resistance of the organism [87,190,191]. In recent years, programmes have been developed to standardise the treatment of SDS [43,83]. In the complex treatment of purulent-necrotic lesions of the lower extremities, rational antibacterial therapy is of great importance [26,45,173,181]. In addition to the choice of antibacterial drugs and their dosage, the ways of antibiotics administration into the patient's body are of great importance [152]. Taking into account the fact that the above-mentioned diseases develop due to circulatory insufficiency in the lower extremities, the ineffectiveness of oral, intramuscular or intravenous administration of drugs becomes clear [63,65]. When drugs are administered intramuscularly or intravenously, due to vascular obliteration [28,49] or due to diabetic micro- and macroangiopathy [51,52], drugs do not reach their destination in the desired concentration. Therefore, intra-arterial administration of drugs is currently used. The method of intra-arterial infusion of drugs proposed in 1935 by Lerish and Fontaine has found wide application in the complex treatment of obliterative diseases of the lower extremities. Practically, this method in the treatment of patients with the most severe limb ischaemia due to endarteritis, atherosclerosis, diabetic angiopathy can be considered the method of choice at present [55].

There are mainly 2 methods of intra-arterial drug administration used:

1). Fractional intra-arterial administration of drugs by repeated arterial punctures;

2). Prolonged intra-arterial catheter therapy [65,66,72], which is performed:

A) catheter insertion directly into the arterial lumen; B) selective probing of aortic branches [22,46];

B) catheter insertion into the lumen of the main artery through its collateral branches [22,63].

The greatest efforts of researchers are focused on the search for drugs for the treatment of wounds in the first phase of the course of purulent-necrotic processes. The effectiveness of wound treatment in this phase largely determines the outcome of the disease as a whole [87]. In this phase, a rapid infectious process unfolds in the wound. Wound microflora maximally manifests its properties: pathogenicity, invasiveness, etc. The wound discharge in this phase is rich in microorganisms, by microbial toxins, enzymes and toxic products of tissue decay [87]. The success of treatment of patients with purulent-necrotic lesions of the lower extremities on the background of DM depends on local treatment [3,34,47]. For this purpose, various antiseptic preparations are used: ointments [23], proteolytic enzymes, adsorbents [87,105], dressings [145], semipermeable membranes [138], and physical methods of treatment. Brummer M et al (2002) used intravenous administration of netilmicin 200mg, gentamicin 120mg, heparin 2500ed, dexamethasone 4mg for 7-10 days and achieved healing of trophic ulcers on the foot [145]. Shaposhnikov V.I. and Zorik V.V. (2001) in the treatment of 38 patients with purulent-necrotic lesions of the lower extremities in DM with the purpose of long-term and permanent suppression of pathogenic microflora placed the affected limb in a double polyethylene bag with 2% boric acid solution [119]. Seliverstov D.V. et al. (1997; 2000) provide a comparative assessment of the clinical efficacy of some combined ointments in the treatment of purulent wounds in patients with DM [105]. According to the authors, combined ointments containing antibiotics and steroidal preparations on polyethylene oxide base have a pronounced antibacterial effect and enhance repair processes.

In recent years, a significant role in the local treatment of purulent-necrotic processes in lower extremities in patients with DM has been assigned to a group of enzymes, including proteolytic enzymes [68,118]. Animal [3,34], bacterial [33,34] proteolytic enzymes are used, of plant [57,84,97] origin. Gostischev V.K. et al. (1996) developed a prolonged form of lidoamidase immobilised on textile cellulose carriers. Prolonged action of the drug up to 24-28 hours was noted [33]. Glyantsev S.P. (1998) cites for clinical comparison the results of treatment of purulent wounds with dalcex-trypsin, trypsin-chlorhexidine wipe, trypsin-urea wipe, profesim, sipralin, gelevin, lysosorb, gentavin [34].

Rakhimov M.R. (2001) studied the pharmacological properties of a domestic enzyme preparation of plant origin - papain [97]. Papain is isolated in pure form from the milky juice of melon tree Carica papaya. It was found that the preparation has high proteolytic activity compared to enzyme preparations of animal and bacterial origin. The disadvantage of papain is its complete loss at low pH levels. At ph - 11, 70% of the drug activity is retained, and at ph - 2.4 papain is completely inactivated [84]. In 1998, employees of the Institute of Chemistry of Plant Substances of the Academy of Sciences of the Republic of Uzbekistan isolated a complex of proteolytic enzymes - cucumazyme - from the milky juice of Carica papaya. Cucumazyme differs from other proteolytic enzymes of animal and plant origin in structural, qualitative and qualitative aspects. quantitative parameters. The preparation is a complex of 5 proteolytic enzymes [papain, a mixture of enzymes known as chymopapain A and B and two highly alkaline proteins peptidases A and B]. When the stability of cucumazyme to ph was investigated, a retention of 40% of its activity was observed even at ph 2.4. The retention of proteolytic activity in a wide range of medium ph and temperature was found, which made it a convenient object for scientific research and practical use [84]. In the complex treatment of purulent-necrotic lesions of the lower extremities, physical methods are widely used - ultraviolet blood irradiation [54,77], laser therapy of wounds [13,17,75,118] and laser blood irradiation [54,78], hyperbaric oxygenation [131,172], ultrasound cavitation of wounds [109,153]. Determining the volume and timing of surgical intervention in DM patients with purulent-necrotic lesions of the lower extremities presents significant difficulties. The volume of surgical intervention depends on the shape, depth, localisation and prevalence of foot lesions, and the presence of osteomyelitis of the foot [23]. The peculiarity of surgical treatment of purulent-necrotic lesions of the foot is a wide opening of the purulent focus with its sanation. Technically correct performance of sanation of the purulent focus, amputation of toes or segments of the foot is extremely important in order to exclude additional tissue trauma and spread of infection. Reconstructive operations on the foot after previous repeated and irrational local surgical interventions without taking into account the anatomical structures of the foot, the form of the lesion, the possibility of subsequent prosthetics, the age and weight of the patient, the course of diabetes and diseases stimulated by it present the greatest difficulty [22]. According to Jung V (1996) and Lepantalo M et al (2000), 83% of high lower limb amputations in patients with diabetes are performed in non-specialised clinics by general surgeons [189,199]. The neuropathic form is mainly treated with dissection and drainage of the fibular spaces [139,168], necrectomy [241,252], disarticulation of the toes, metatarsal resections [218], amputations of the tibia and femur, and skin flap transplantation [19,220]. In progressive purulent-necrotic processes in the lower extremities against the background of diabetes mellitus almost the only surgical intervention is amputation of the lower limb at the thigh level, the number of which reaches 30-50% [10,16,187]. Chur N.N. et al. (2000) consider the following indications for high primary amputation in SDS patients: uncorrectable ischaemia and impossibility of its correction by surgery; progressive wet gangrene of the foot with spread of the process to the lower leg; threat of septic condition development in purulent-necrotic phlegmon of the foot [118].

CLINICAL MATERIAL AND METHODS RESEARCH

Characterisation of clinical material

352 patients with purulent-necrotic lesions of the lower limbs against the background of diabetes mellitus were examined.
The patients were divided into 4 groups depending on the treatment performed:
Group I - 112 patients who underwent traditional complex treatment including correction of carbohydrate, protein, fat metabolism, rheological properties of blood, improvement of microcirculatory channel, antibiotic therapy, treatment of concomitant pathologies;
II group - 83 patients with purulent-necrotic lesions of the lower limbs against the background of diabetes mellitus, who underwent complex treatment with local application of cucumazyme;
III group - 95 patients in whom local application of cucumazyme and ultrasound cavitation of wounds were included in the complex of treatment measures;
IV group - 62 patients who received local application of cucumazyme, ultrasound cavitation of wounds and autotransfusion of ultraviolet irradiated blood (AUVOC).
Type I DM occurred in 23 patients, type II DM in 329 patients. The age of patients ranged from 17 to 84 years, the average age was 62.7 years. More often purulent necrotic lesions occurred at the age of 45-74 years.
Patients in all groups were distributed according to the WHO and Wagner (1979) classification. The WHO classification includes distribution of patients depending on clinical forms - neuropathic, ischaemic and mixed. As can be seen from the table, neuropathic and mixed (neuroischaemic) forms of diabetic foot syndrome prevailed in all groups of patients, which corresponds to the literature data. The ischaemic form was found in 24 patients (6.8%). The osteoarthropathic form of DFS was found in 62 patients (17.6%).

Distribution of patients with SDS according to WHO classification.

Shape	Group I	Group 2	Group 3	Group 4	Total
Neuropathic	62(55,3%)	43(51,8%)	44(46,3%)	36(58%)	185(52,6%)
Osteoarthropathy	16(14,3%)	12(14,5%)	24(25,3%)	10(16,2%)	62(17,6%)
Ischaemic	7(6,3)	6(7,2%)	6(6,3%)	5(8%)	24(6,8%)
Mixed	27(24,1%)	22(26,5%)	21(22,1%)	11(17,8%)	81(23%)
Total	112(100%)	83(100%)	95(100%)	62(100%)	352(100%)

Distribution of patients with SDS according to the Wagner classification

Degrees	Group I	Group II	Group III	Group IV	Total
0-degree	10 (8,9%)	7 (8,4%)	6 (6,4%)	5 (8%)	28 (7,9%)
I-II degree	23 (20,5%)	16 (19,3%)	20 (21%)	14 (22,7%)	73 (20,7%)
III degree	31 (27,7%)	22 (26,5%)	29 (30,5%)	18 (29%)	100 (28,5%)
IV degree	39 (34,8%)	30 (36,1%)	31 (32,6%)	20 (32,4%)	120 (34,1%)
V degree.	9 (8,1%)	8 (9,7%)	9 (9,5%)	5 (8%)	31 (8,8%)
Total	112 (100%)	83 (100%)	95 (100%)	62 (100%)	352 (100%)

When distributing patients according to Wagner, the depth and prevalence of purulent-necrotic process were taken into account, including 5 stages.

Characterisation of the research methods

Rheovasography (RVG) and ultrasound Doppler ultrasonography (USDG) were performed to study blood flow in the lower extremities.

RVG was performed using a 4-RG-1A apparatus. The following leads were used to record rheograms of the lower limbs: longitudinal rheography of the tibia (circular electrodes were placed on the proximal and distal parts of the tibia) and rheography of the foot (proximal electrode was located in the lower third of the tibia, distal electrode - on the I toe of the foot). The curves were decoded using parallel recorded electro- and phonocardiograms and differential rheogram reflecting the rate of change of the studied process in time. Analysis of rheograms included quantitative characterisation. Quantitative analysis included calculation of amplitude, time and velocity parameters of the curve - rheovasographic index (RI).

USDG was performed on an Aloka (Japan) device equipped with a Doppler attachment. When analysing spectrograms, attention was paid to changes in the maximum blood flow velocity (Max A) and peripheral resistance index of the vascular wall (RP).

Ankle-shoulder index (ASI) was determined by the formula ASI= ankle systolic BP/shoulder systolic BP.

In the norm, the LPI was equal to 1.0. Below 0.9 was characteristic of decreased blood flow in the lower limb.

Echoosteometry was performed using the Echoostemometer EOM-1ts device. The ultrasound conductivity of the metatarsal, tibia, radius and clavicle bones was studied. The obtained results were given in m/s.

Chemical analysis of bone tissue. Bone tissues removed during the operation were ozolised and the content of lead, zinc, phosphorus, calcium was determined using the titrimetric method. The obtained results were expressed in µg/g and in

%.

Morphological studies of biopsy specimens taken from patients with diabetes mellitus complicated by purulent-necrotic processes of the lower extremities were performed in the traditional way, in particular, the slices were fixed in 10% neutral formalin solution. Histological sections taken from paraffin blocks were stained with hematoxylin-eosin and viewed with a light microscope "Biolam-16".

Microbiological studies. Aerobic microflora was isolated by Birger M.O. method by sowing the wound discharge on nutrient media (blood and milk-yolk-salt agar). The sowing was incubated in the thermostat at 37C for 24 hours. If microbial association was detected, all grown colonies were identified, the predominant flora was identified and its sensitivity to antibiotics was determined using the disc method. The isolation and identification of anaerobic non-spore-forming gram-negative bacteria was performed by the method of V.I. Kocherovets in accordance with the methodological recommendations of the Ministry of Health of the RSFSR of 1984. "Microbiological diagnostics of bacteroid infection in surgery". Cultivation of anaerobes was performed in microanaerostats with a palladium catalyst filled with a gas mixture consisting of hydrogen -10%, carbon dioxide -10% and nitrogen 80%, stimulating the growth of many species of anaerobic non-spore-forming Gram-negative bacteria. Primary cultures were viewed after 2 days and further every 1-2 days. The duration of cultivation in the absence of growth was at least 7 days. Quantitative assessment of bacterial infestation of purulent wounds was performed according to the Baxter method modified by M.I. Kuzin et al. (119).
Quantification of the grown colonies in different dilutions was calculated CFU/g.

Immunological methods. To investigate the immune status we used monoclonal antibodies produced by the Institute of Immunology of the Russian Federation: to determine T-lymphocytes (SD-5) - LT1; helper-inducer subpopulation - LT4; suppressor cytotoxic killers (SD-8) - LT8; B-lymphocytes - 3F-3.

The pool of "null" lymphocytes was determined by the indirect method according to Froland et al (1973) by subtracting the sum of the number of T- and B-cells from the total number of lymphocytes.

Immunoglobulins of class A, M and G were determined by radial immunodiffusion according to Mancini (1964).

The phagocytic index of immunity was determined using a one-day culture of Staphylococcus aureus.

The agar diffusion method was used to determine serum lysozyme levels (119).

Neurological examinations. Clinical investigation of the severity of diabetic neuropathy consisted of two parts: a) assessment of symptoms (paresthesias, burning, numbness, pain) and b) clinical neurological examination using quantitative tests (6).

Tactile (using monofilament or cotton wool), pain (using a neuropen or gear wheel), vibration (using a tuning box) and temperature sensitivities were studied.

Characterisation and technique of local application of the proteolytic enzyme cucumazyme.

Cucumazyme is a total proteolytic enzyme preparation of plant origin, obtained by employees of the Institute of Chemistry of Plant Substances, Academy of Sciences of the Republic of Uzbekistan from melon tree Carica Papaya. Clinical approbation of cucumazyme was carried out with our participation. The drug is registered by the Main Department of Control quality of medicines and medical equipment of the MH RUz, registration certificate No. 98/331/2. Permission for use in practical medicine was issued by the order of the MH RUz №331 dated 06 July 1998. The drug has proteolytic activity of a wide range of action. Enzymes papain, chymopapain and three proteinase enzymes belonging to sulfhydryl group of proteinases are the active ingredients of the drug. Cucumazyme, unlike other proteolytic enzymes, has pronounced proteolytic, fibrinolytic, chondrolytic and anti-inflammatory actions. When studying the stability of proteinases in the zone of pH 2.5-11, it was found that cucumazyme is stable in the interval of pH 6-9. Significant stability of the drug was maintained at alkaline pH values. Thus, at pH 11.0, 70% of the activity was retained. However, even at pH 2.4, up to 40% of activity was retained. The complex preparation cucumazyme in this respect favourably differed from pure papain, which was completely inactivated (132). Resistance to high temperatures, urea and other denaturing agents, and a greater depth of protein hydrolysis contributed to the wide use of the preparation in practice.

Cucumazyme was applied topically at a dose of 10mg. (50 proteolytic units). The drug was dissolved in 10 ml of 0.5% novocaine solution before use. The technique of local application of the drug was as follows: after opening of the purulent focus and necrectomy the wounds were loosely filled with a turunda soaked in cucumazyme solution. Besides, deep wounds, fistulas were washed with cucumazyme solution through a microirrigator. Dressings were performed daily until the wound was completely cleared of purulent-necrotic masses and granulation appeared.

Methodology of ultrasonic examination.

USC was performed with the URSK-8T apparatus at the vibration amplitude of 0.55-0.60 μm, resonance frequency of 26.12-28.85 kHz and total exposure of 10-12 minutes. USC was performed from the first day of the purulent centre opening. Purulent cavities were filled with 10mg of cucumazyme dissolved in 5ml of 0.5% novocaine solution and ultrasound was applied at a distance of 0.5-1cm from the wound wall. In the presence of superficial, extensive areas of necrosis, the limb was placed in a tray with cucumazyme solution and ultrasound sounding was performed. Ultrasound was performed for 10-12 minutes. The number of sessions varied from 5 to 9 times.

Methodology for conducting AUFOC.

Under aseptic conditions, blood was drawn from the elbow vein of the patient in the amount of 1.5-2ml per kg of the patient's weight, which is 120-150ml. Blood was taken into a vial with haemoconservative "Glugitsir" or 50ml of 0.9% sodium chloride solution, where 1ml-5000 U of heparin solution was added. Reverse transfusion of blood was performed immediately after collection. Ultraviolet irradiation of blood was performed by "UFOC" apparatus equipped with mercury-quartz lamp "DRT-8" during blood collection and reverse transfusion. AUVOC was performed daily, on average 4-5 sessions per course of treatment. The degree of compensated DM, clinical form, prevalence and depth of necrotic process lesion, presence of concomitant pathology determined the treatment tactics.

The traditional set of therapeutic measures included:

-correction of glycaemia and glucosuria;

-correction of ischaemic disorders: improvement of blood rheological properties, correction of coagulopathy under control of coagulogram indicators;

-detoxification tonic therapy (haemodez, infusion of electrolytes, protein preparations, plasma and blood);

-targeted antibiotic therapy taking into account microbiological studies;

-local treatment - proteolytic enzymes, water-soluble polyethylene oxide ointments;

-discharge of the lower limb - temporary (restriction of movement, rest, prescription of bed rest, plaster cast) and long-term - wearing orthopaedic shoes;

-operative intervention;

-treatment of concomitant pathologies.

RESULTS OF COMPLEX TREATMENT OF DIABETIC FOOT SYNDROME

The complex of therapeutic measures in purulent-necrotic complications of the lower extremities against the background of diabetes mellitus should be aimed at the correction of the most important pathogenetic links of the diabetic foot syndrome. Treatment of infected lesions of the feet was carried out taking into account the form of the lesion, prevalence infection, presence osteomyelitis of the foot, which dictated the choice of tactics of podiatric or surgical management. In this chapter, we highlighted the results of complex treatment of SDS using cucumazyme, USC and AUVOC. We present the results of the study the influence of a new proteolytic enzyme of plant origin with a complex composition - cucumazyme and physical methods (ultrasound, AUVOC) on the course of purulent-necrotic processes of the lower extremities in SDS, taking into account the clinical forms and stages of SDS. The treatment results were confirmed by the data of clinical, instrumental, microbiological and immunomorphological studies.

Results of traditional complex treatment of purulent-necrotic complications of lower limbs in diabetes mellitus

Traditional complex treatment was performed in 112 patients with purulent necrotic complications of the lower extremities against the background of diabetes mellitus (stage 0-10, stage I-II-23, stage III-31, stage IV-39, stage V-9). Neuropathic form of diabetic foot was found in 62, osteoarthropathic in 16, ischaemic in 7 and mixed in 27 patients. Improvement of the general condition on the background of the conducted complex therapy was observed in 72% of patients. Dull, diffuse pain in the extremities, arising mainly at rest and decreasing with physical activity, which are characteristic of distal sensorimotor neuropathy, were completely eliminated only in 62% of patients.

Results of clinical examination of SDS patients under traditional complex treatment.

Clinical signs	Result
Improvement of general condition	72%
Disappearance of the burning sensation	74%
Reduction in diffuse pain	69%
Disappearance of numbness in the limb	58%
Disappearance of painful cramps in the limb	42%
Lengthening the distance travelled without pain	33%

Paresthesias, characterised by sensation tingling, "buzzing." "burning" sensations disappeared in 74% of patients. Sensations of numbness of distal limbs disappeared in 58% of patients. Painful cramps in limbs after complex traditional treatment were relieved in 42% of patients. The results of complex treatment of patients with neuroischaemic form of diabetic foot (34 patients) were of particular interest. Significant clinical improvement was noted in 12 patients with a mild form of ischemia, which was manifested in the disappearance of pain at rest, normalisation of the skin colour of the feet, improvement of well-being (normalisation of sleep and appetite). The distance walked without pain lengthened to 300-400 metres. Reduction of ischaemia stage by clinical signs was noted in 12 patients (35.3%). In 3 patients with a mild form of the disease compensation of carbohydrate metabolism came as a result of diet and nutrition without insulin therapy. In the absence of glycaemic compensation in severe diabetes 7 patients were prescribed short-acting insulin 18-36 units per day. B vitamins, ascorbic and nicotinic acids, retabolil were used in complex treatment, and concomitant diseases were treated. Normalisation of blood sugar level in these patients came on the 5th-6th day. At severe degree of diabetes (decompensation stage), especially in the presence of purulent-necrotic process in the extremities, high hyperglycaemia up to 9,1±0,75 mmol/l and glucosuria 3% and higher were observed. In these cases a combination of short- and long-acting insulin was administered from the first day of admission to the clinic in order to compensate diabetes. As it is known, in purulent-necrotic lesions of the foot in patients with diabetes mellitus, there is a syndrome of mutual aggravation, i.e. the level of glycaemia as well as other clinical manifestations are directly proportional to the severity of purulent-necrotic process. Therefore, even against the background of large doses of insulin, the level of glycaemia was on high figures and tended to decrease only after liquidation of necrotic focus. Therefore, high glycaemia in these patients was estimated by us not as insufficiency of exogenously administered insulin dose, but as a manifestation of the syndrome of mutual aggravation. On the average decrease of glycaemia level was observed on the 7th-8th day after liquidation of purulent-necrotic process up to 8,3±0,3 mmol/l ($p>0,05$). At instrumental investigations the following was observed. An unreliable increase of RI up to 0.57±0.014 ($p>0.05$) was observed on RVG (Fig. 4.1.1.).The USDG also showed a non-significant increase in Max A from 17.58 ± 0.5cm/s to 19.45 ± 0.78cm/s ($p>0.05$). PLI increased from 0.89 ± 0.02 to 0.92 ± 0.029 ($p>0.05$), indicating a slight improvement in blood supply in the limb (Fig.1). The study of coagulation system parameters at the patients' admission to the clinic showed the presence of hypercoagulable state: PTI 99,2±2,3%, fibrinogen 6,075±0,28g/l.

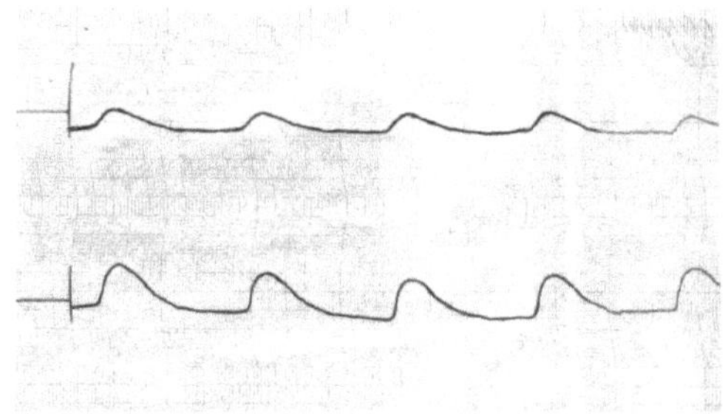

Fig. 1. RVG of the patient on the background of traditional therapy.

On the background of traditional treatment there was a tendency to decrease PTI up to 96±2%, and fibrinogen on the contrary increased up to 6,51±0,6 g/l (p>0,05). Thus, the results of our studies showed that against the background of traditional complex therapy there is some improvement of blood flow in the lower extremities, although to unreliable figures.

Indicators of instrumental and laboratory studies of patients receiving conventional therapy.

Indicators	Before treatment	After treatment
LPI	0,89±0,02	0,92±0,029
RI	0,55±0,01	0,57±0,014
MaxA cm/s	17,58±0,5	19,45±0,78
PTI%	99,2±2,25	96±2
Fibrinogen g/l	6,075±0,28	6,51±0,6
Blood glucose mmol/l	9,1±0,75	8,3±0,3
Glucose in urine %	3±0,2*	1±0,1*

Note: *-p<0.05 compared to before treatment.

Surgical interventions were avoided in 39 patients. Seventy-three patients (65.2%), mostly with stages III-IV-V of diabetic foot syndrome, underwent surgical interventions. The study of the course of local manifestations of diabetic foot showed positive efficacy of traditional therapy in 37 patients (33%). Disappearance of clinical manifestations was observed in 5 patients with 0-stage, 2 patients showed improvement of the condition. And only in 3 patients the condition remained unchanged.

Twenty-three patients with I-II stages of SDS had ulcerative defects on the foot, who were mainly treated with local therapy. In the alteration phase, solutions of liquid antiseptics (1% solution of dioxidine, iodopyrone) were used to prevent the infectious process.

Treatment indices of the patients of the first group.

Indicators	0	I-II	III	IV	V	Total
Total number of patients	10 (8,9%)	23 (20,5%)	31 (27,7%)	39 (34,8%)	9 (8,1%)	112 (100%)
Operated on	-	-	27 (87,1%)	39 (100%)	7 (77,8%)	73 (65,2%)
Cf. bed day	-	-	31,4±1,9	30,3±1,2	65,2±3,8	34±1,5
P/o complications	-	-	-	7 (17,9%)	6 (85,7%)	13 (17,8%)
P/o lethality	-	-	1 (3,7%)	4 (10,3%)	2 (28,6%)	7 (9,6%)
Not operated on	10 (100%)	23 (100%)	4 (12,1%)	-	2 (22,2%)	39 (34,8%)
Lethality	-	-	-	4	2	6(5,4%)
Total mortality	-	-	1 (3,2%)	8 (20,5%)	4 (44,4%)	13 (17,8%)

After the transition of the alteration phase to the exudation phase, ointments made on the basis of polyethylene glycol (Levomekol, dioxidine ointment) were applied. Clearing of the surface of trophic ulcers from purulent-fibrinous masses was observed on average on 12.1 ± 0.25 days. Reduction of ulcer size was slow. The appearance of granulation tissue was observed on 14.7 ± 0.3 days. Healing of trophic ulcers was observed in 11 patients. In other 12 patients trophic ulcers decreased in size, signs of inflammation were eliminated. Average terms of treatment with I-II stages were 17,5 days. No surgical interventions were performed in patients with 0-I-II stages of SDS. 73 patients (65.2%) with III-IV-V stages of SDS underwent surgical interventions.

In 4 patients with stage III with neuropathic form on the background of traditional treatment the suppression of purulent-necrotic process was noted. 27 out of 31 patients with stage III SDS underwent surgical interventions and 43 operations were performed in total. 14 patients (with neuropathy - 7, osteoarthropathy - 3, mixed form - 4) with phlegmon of the foot were opened on the day of admission. In this case we used a "club-shaped" incision, cutting out skin-fascial flaps (Fig. 2.). This incision allows to perform radical excision of necrotic tissues. Staged necrectomies were performed in 12 patients against the background of the therapy. Separation of purulent-necrotic process in this group was observed in 15 patients (with neuropathy - 10, osteoarthropathy - 3, mixed form - 2) who underwent organ-preserving operations. Finger disarticulations were performed in 4 cases. In 1 patient, considering the combined lesion of II-III-IV toes, Sharpe's amputation of the foot was performed. The wounds were open, dressings were made 2 times a day until granulation appeared, and then daily or once in 2 days. Wounds after opening of pustules were loosely filled with turundas, moistened with a solution of proteolytic enzymes. At the stage of wound cleansing from purulent-necrotic masses, hydrophilic ointments were applied.

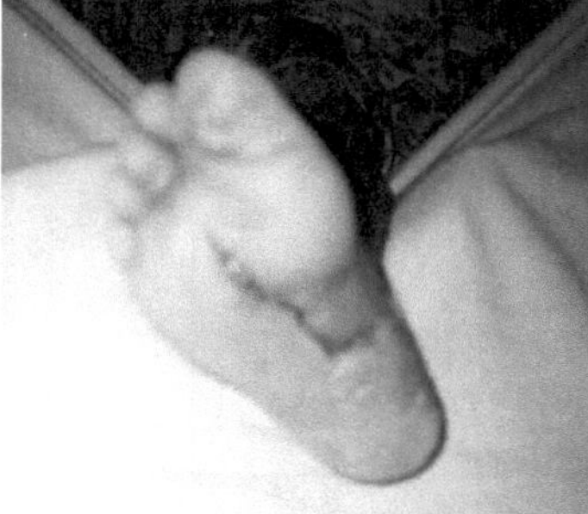

Fig. 2. View of the wound after opening phlegmon of the right foot.

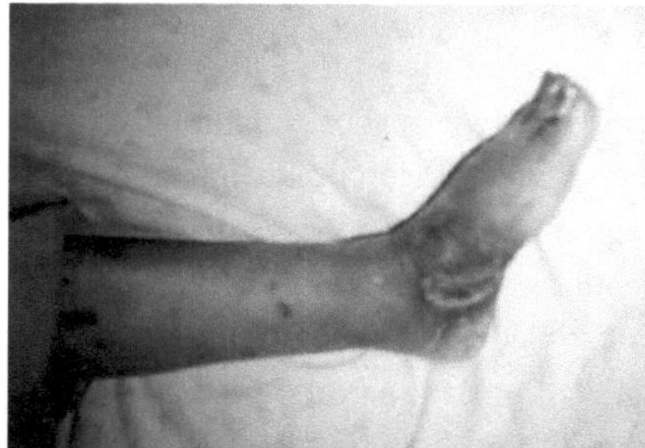

Figure 3. Incorrectly performed incision for opening phlegmon of the foot.

In 12 patients (with neuropathy-5, ischaemia-1, osteoarthropathy-2, mixed form-4), taking into account the progression of purulent-necrotic process, high thigh amputations were performed. The reason of spreading of necrotic process in 4 patients was different incisions used for opening of plantar phlegmon of the foot, which did not provide sufficiently radical removal of necrotic tissues. In 1 patient with ischaemia there was a contraindication to reconstructive vascular surgery after consultation of an angiosurgeon. In 7 cases, after a short-term subsidence of inflammation, the necrotic process resumption was observed. In the postoperative period 1 patient died due to cardiovascular insufficiency. Average terms of treatment of patients with stage III SDS were 31,4±1,9 days. All 39 patients of the first group with stage IV SDS were operated on. Separation of the necrotic process was noted in 38 patients (22 with neuropathy, 5 with osteoarthropathy, 11 with mixed form), who underwent finger disarticulation in 30 cases and necrectomy in 8 cases. The most severe contingent were patients with gangrene of the I toe of the foot (8 patients). These 8 patients (with neuropathy-5, osteoarthropathy-1, mixed form-2), after disarticulation of fingers, taking into account the spread of necrotic process, performed Sharpe and Lisfranc amputations of the foot, which were ineffective and they were subsequently forced to undergo amputations at the thigh level. Primary thigh amputation was performed in 1 patient with critical limb ischaemia. The lethal outcome was observed in 4 cases (increasing cardiovascular and renal-hepatic insufficiency in 3 patients, progression of necrosis of the femoral stump in 1 patient). The average treatment period was 30.3±1.2 days. In 1 patient with stage V neuropathic SDS, conventional treatment was able to isolate the purulent-necrotic process and preserve the supporting function of the foot. Hip amputations were performed in 6 cases due to progression of purulent-necrotic process. 4 patients died - 2 before the operation due to multiorgan failure, 2 after the operation on the background of cardiovascular insufficiency. The average treatment period was 65.2 days.On the background of traditional therapy microbial susceptibility remained above critical figures even on the 5th day of treatment, amounting to 3.2x10 -10^{57}

Microbiological investigations during conventional treatment.

Patient group	Microbial contamination of 1g of tissue.			
	Twenty-four hours			
	1	3	5	9
Conventional treatment	5.1x10 -8 1010	4.5x10 -7 108	3.2x10 -5 107	2,8x104- 105

In group I patients, where traditional complex therapy was performed, microbial growth was detected in 72% of patients with microbial contamination of 1g of wound tissue 2.1x10 -10^{34} . Absence of microbial growth was noted in 28% of cases.

Microbiological investigations in SDS at the end of treatment.

Patient group	Microbial growth %	Microbial contamination 1g of tissue	Absence of Microbial growth %
Conventional treatment	72%	2,1x103 -104	28%

The results of traditional treatment were confirmed by immunomorphological studies. The improvement of immunological reactivity in the course of treatment was one of the reliable indicators of the reduction of the inflammatory process in the lower limb. In immunological studies in this group of patients there was an unreliable increase in the content of T-lymphocytes, T-helpers ($p>0.05$), but the deficit of T-lymphocytes compared to normal values was 15%. Absolute and relative indices of B lymphocytes still remained in significantly high figures, being 477,9 ± 22,9 kl/μl and 25,4±1,1% respectively (p<0,05).

Immunity indices of the I group of patients at the end of treatment.

Indicators	Before treatment	At the end of the treatment
T-lymphocytes %	1057,7±38,3 48,3±3,2	1030±36,4 49,7±2,1
T-helper cells %	680,5±36,6 23,2±3	651,9±44,6 25,3±2,4
T-suppressors %	375,5±41,7 17±1	375,3±29,6 17,1±0,7
B-lymphocytes %	326,8±22,5 22±0,66	477,9±22,9* 25,4±1,1*
0-lymphocytes %	434,7±45,5 29,7±3	434,9±67,4 24,9±3,3
Phagocytic count %	43±3,5	46,9±3,9
Ig A g/l	1,1±0,04	1,1±0,03
Ig M g/l	3,6±0,3	3,2±0,3
Ig G g/l	13,6±0,7	13,5±0,5
Lysozyme mg%	1,3±0,2	1,6±0,2

Note: * - p<0.05. in relation to baseline values.

There was also an unreliably high content of 0 lymphocytes 434,9±67,4 kl/μl and 24,9±3,3% (p>0,01), which showed the insufficient formation of cellular immunity to the existing purulent-necrotic processes in the lower limb. When studying the indices of humoral immunity it was noted that even at the end of treatment the content of immunoglobulins of class M and G were in unreliably high figures - 13,6 ± 0,7 and 3,6 ± 0,3 (p>0,01). The content of lysozyme in blood serum was still low 1.63 ± 0.24 (p>0.01).At traditional methods of treatment of purulent-necrotic wounds of patients with diabetes mellitus in cytological preparations the presence of neutrophils, macrophages, detritus masses was noted, in histological sections necrotic tissue among elements of skin and subcutaneous tissue is also revealed.

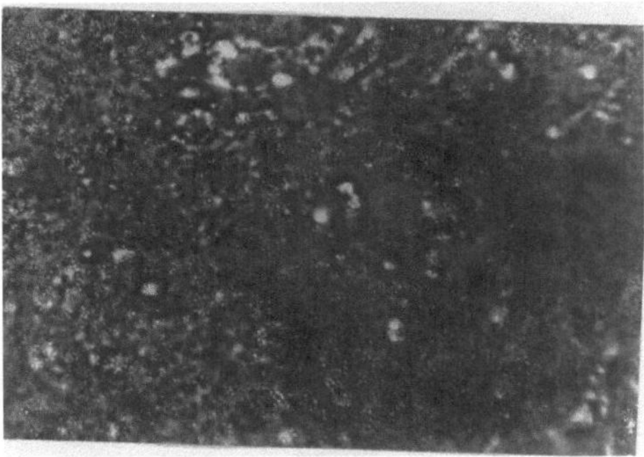

Figure 4. Presence of neutrophils, macrophages, detrital masses in the smears of prints. Light microscopy. Haematoxylin-eosin staining. Eq.x160.

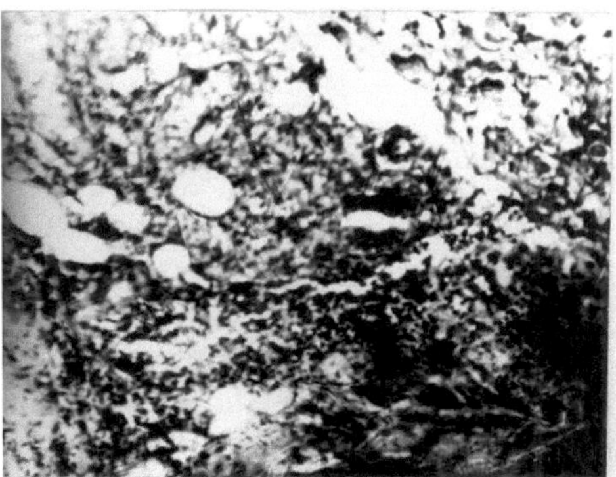

Fig. 5. Skin with subcutaneous tissue with detrital mass, elements of inflammation in traditional treatment. Light microscopy. Haematoxylin-eosin staining. Eq.x160.

Thus, 39 patients (34.8%) managed to stop the purulent-necrotic process against the background of traditional treatment. 27 patients (23.7%) underwent femoral amputation, and in 46 (41.1%) patients the surgical interventions were organ-preserving.

Results of complex treatment of SDS with the use of cucumazyme.

Out of 83 patients of the second group with neuropathic form of diabetic foot were 43 patients, osteoarthropathy 12, ischaemic 6 and mixed form was found in 22 patients. In order to correct hyperglycaemia, 24 patients were prescribed sugar-lowering drugs in tablet form, the remaining 59 patients were switched to short-acting insulin. Blood glucose on admission of patients with neuropathic and osteoarthropathic forms to the hospital was within 8.7 ± 0.85 mmol/l. By the end of treatment there was an unreliable decrease in glucose concentration to 7.4 ± 0.4 mmol/l ($p>0.05$). Normalisation of glycaemic index was accompanied by improvement of clinical manifestations of neuropathy. Improvement of general condition was observed in 94% of patients. Dull, diffuse pain in the extremities, arising mainly at rest and decreasing with physical activity, which are characteristic of distal sensorimotor neuropathy were completely eliminated in 96% of patients Paresthesias characterised by tingling, "buzzing" sensation,"burning" after treatment disappeared in 92% of patients. Sensations of numbness of distal limbs were not observed in 89% of patients. Painful cramps in the extremities were eliminated in 84% of patients.

Results of clinical examination of group II patients.

Clinical signs	Result
Improvement of general condition	94,5%
Disappearance of the burning sensation	92%
Reduction in diffuse pain	85%
Disappearance of numbness in the limb	89%
Disappearance of painful cramps in the limb	84%
Distance extension passable without pain	48%

If the osteoarthropathic form prevailed and destructive processes were present, plaster casts were applied before and after surgical interventions to relieve the limb. 28 patients with ischaemic and mixed forms of diabetic foot received vascular therapy in complex treatment.

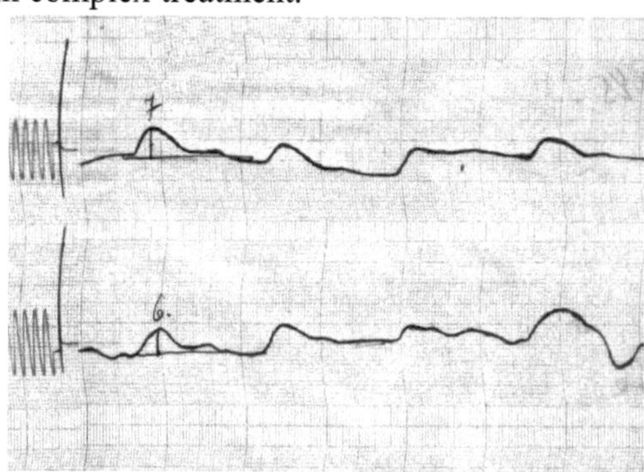

Figure 6. RVG score before treatment.

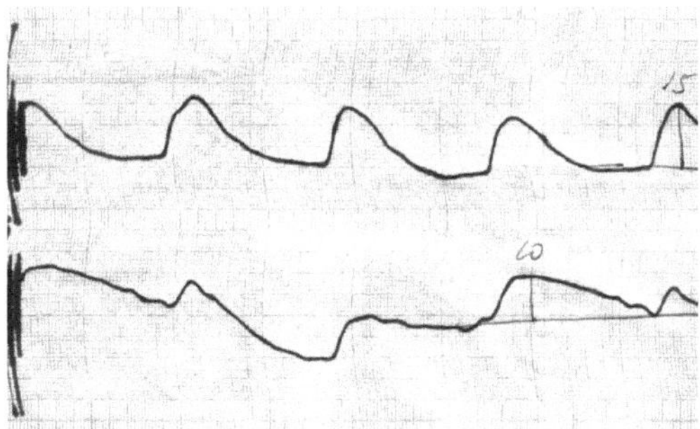

Figure 7. RVG score by the end of treatment.

Complete disappearance of pain syndrome was observed in 24 patients, significant reduction of pain in the limb was observed in 10 patients. Especially pronounced effect was observed in patients with I-II III stages of ischaemia. Pain-free walking distance of more than 500 metres was observed in 24 patients. Clinical effect was achieved in 26 patients (94,5%). The effectiveness of treatment was also confirmed by the data of instrumental studies. Significant changes indicating the improvement of blood flow in the lower limb were obtained when determining the LPI. There was an increase in LPI up to 1.04 ± 0.018 ($p<0.05$). On rheovasograms at the end of the treatment the increase of RI up to 0.60±0.002 ($p<0.05$) was clearly revealed, which indicated the restoration of the main type of blood flow in the lower limb. This was also confirmed by USDG findings - there was a significant increase in MaxA up to19.4±0.3 cm/s ($p<0.05$).

Indicators of instrumental and laboratory studies in group II patients.

Indicators	Before treatment	After treatment
LPI	0,94±0,01	1,04±0,018*
RI	0,57±0,008	0,6±0,002*
MaxA m/s	18±0,3	19,4±0,3*
PTI%	98,22±2,6	86,44±2,7*
Fibrinogen g/l	5,18±0,44	4,3±0,3
Blood sugar mmol/l	8,7±0,85	7,4±0,4
Sugar in the urine	More than 3 per cent	

Note: *-$p<0.05$ compared to before treatment.

23 patients (7 with stage 0, 14 with stage I-II and 2 with stage V) underwent conservative measures. In the treatment of 16 patients with stage I-II diabetic foot, where there were superficial and deep trophic ulcers along with complex conservative therapy, the main emphasis was on local treatment (Fig. 8). From the first day of the patients' admission to the clinic the proteolytic enzyme of

plant origin cucumazyme was applied locally at 50 PE (proposal No. 2082). Antibiotic therapy was not applied to these patients. On the 3-4 day the surface of trophic ulcers was cleared from purulent-fibrinous plaque, on the 5-6 day granulation tissue appeared.

Treatment indicators of the patients of the second group.

Indicators	0	I-II	III	IV	V	Total
Total number of patients	7	16	22	30	8	83 (100%)
Operated on	-	2	22	30	6	60 (72,3%)
Cf. bed day	-	13,5±1	18,9±1	26,2±1,2	24,1±1,5	23,7±1,2
P/o complications	-	-	-	-	1	1(1,6%)
Not operated on	7	14	-	-	2	23 (27,7%)
Cf. bed day	14,2	15,7	-	-	32	16,6±

Complete healing of trophic ulcers was observed in 14 patients (87.5%) on an average of 10.7 ± 0.3 days (Fig. 9). The remaining 2 patients with trophic ulcers of the toes on the background of destructive osteoarthropathy underwent finger disarticulation. The average treatment time for patients with stage I-II was 13.5 days.In the second group, 60 (72.3%) patients underwent surgical interventions. In 2 patients with trophic ulcers, despite the absence of In patients with visible inflammatory processes in the foot (stage I-II), the EOM showed a decrease in sound conduction of phalangeal bones less than 2500m/s, who were diagnosed with destructive osteoarthropathy. These patients underwent finger disarticulation.

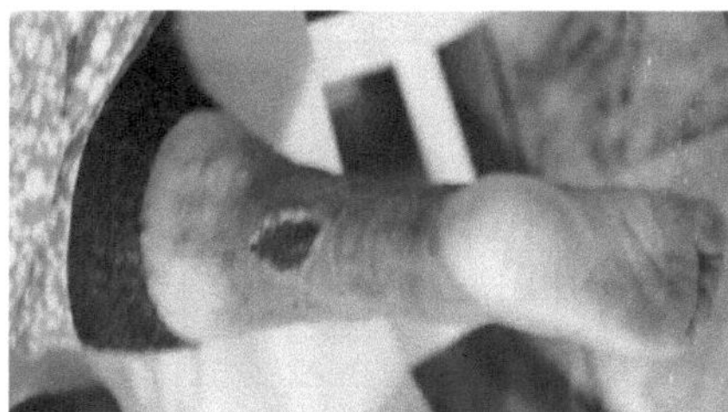

Figure 8. View of trophic ulcer of the tibia before treatment.

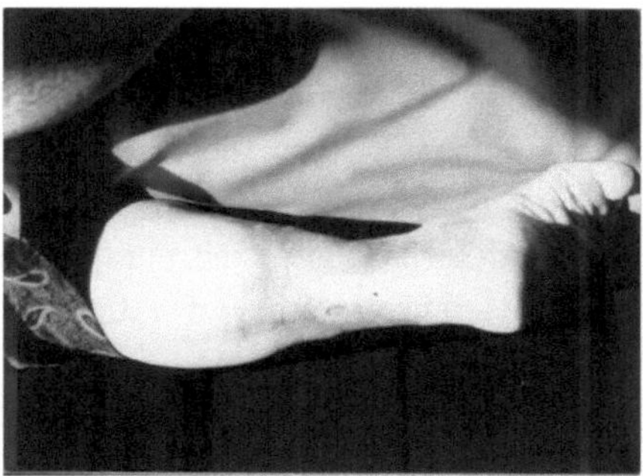

Fig. 9. View of trophic ulcer of the same patient on the 9th day of treatment Cucumazyme.

All 22 patients (with neuropathy - 12, ischaemia - 1, osteoarthropathy - 3, mixed form - 6) underwent surgical interventions with stage III and a total of 29 operations. 11 patients with phlegmon of the foot were performed open purulent foci. Subsequently, they underwent necrectomies in the course of dressings. 2 patients (with neuropathy-1, osteoarthropathy-1) due to involvement in the purulent-necrotic process were performed disarticulation of fingers. The wounds were loosely filled with turundas and napkins soaked in cucumazyme solution. The time of wounds clearing from purulent-necrotic tissues was observed at 9.7±0.3 days. By 10,7±0,3 days.wounds began to be filled with granulation tissue. In 5 patients the wound defect was closed by transplantation of a free skin flap according to Tirsch. Average terms of treatment of patients with stage III were 18,9±1,0 days. All patients managed to preserve the supporting function of the foot by the treatment.A total of 41 surgical interventions were performed in 30 patients with stage IV SDS. Wet gangrene of fingers and feet occurred in 18 patients, dry gangrene in 12 patients. Gangrene on the basis of neuropathy occurred in 14, osteoarthropathy in 12, ischaemia in 2, mixed form in 3 patients. Gangrene of the I toe was observed in 10 patients, in the other 20 patients the necrotic process affected the II-V toes of the foot. Local therapy consisted in application of cucumazyme. 1 patient with ischaemic form, after consultation of a vascular surgeon, was referred to the department of vascular surgery for reconstructive surgery on the main arteries of the limb. In 9 patients with wet gangrene of fingers using cucumazyme it was possible to stop inflammatory process around necrosis, to transfer wet gangrene to dry necrosis. Subsequently, staged necrectomies were independent operations in this category of patients. After delimitation of the necrotic process, 19 patients underwent disarticulation of the toes with removal of flexor tendons. In 4 of them, taking into account the destructive form of osteoarthropathy, the operation was supplemented by removal of the head of the corresponding metatarsal bones. In 2 patients with neuropathic form, due to the progression of necrosis after disarticulation of the toes, Sharpe's amputation of the foot was subsequently performed. The local application of cucumazyme allowed on the average 9.7 ± 0.3 days after the operation to clear the wound surface from the purulent layer. In 2 cases the wound defect was closed by transplantation of a free skin flap according to Tirsch.

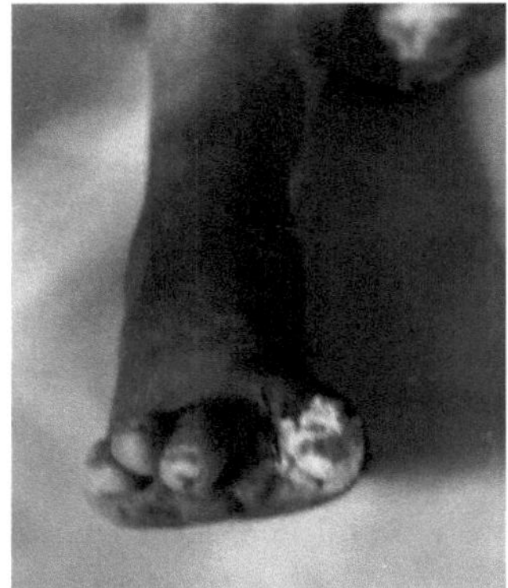

Figure 10. Granulating wound after disarticulation of the first finger.

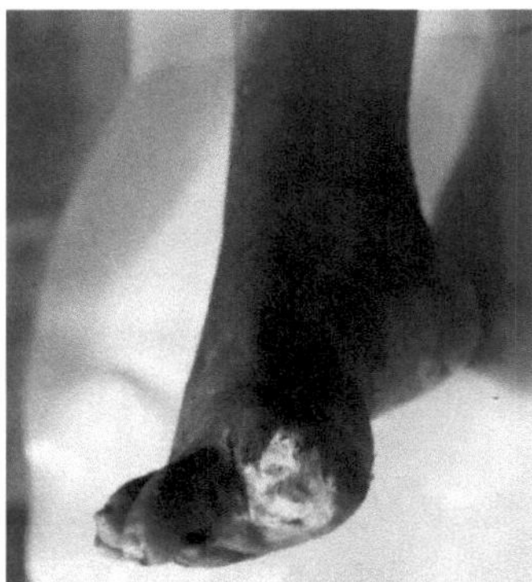

Figure 11. Closed wound defects by skin grafting according to Tiersch.

Given the progression of the purulent-necrotic process, 7 patients (with neuropathy-3, ischaemia-1 and mixed form-3) underwent femoral amputation. Of them 5 patients underwent primary thigh amputation on the next day of their admission to the clinic due to severe septic condition on vital indications. No postoperative complications were observed. The average period of treatment was 26.2±1.0 days.

The best results were obtained in the treatment of patients with stage V. On the background of cucumazyme application on the 7th-8th day of treatment we managed to stop the inflammatory process in 2 patients. Swelling and hyperaemia of the foot disappeared, it became possible to determine a clear demarcation boundary. 1 patient due to destructive form of osteoarthropathy underwent disarticulation of the II-III toe with removal of the metatarsal bone head. 5 patients (3 with neuropathy, 1 with osteoarthropathy, 1 with mixed form) underwent foot amputation after suppression of purulent inflammatory process. Due to the progression of gangrenous process 1 patient with ischaemic form underwent thigh amputation with fatal outcome after the operation against the background of growing cardiovascular insufficiency. The average treatment period was 24.1±1.2 days.In microbiological studies on the background of cucumazyme reliable reduction of microbial contamination was observed on the 3rd day of treatment to 3.1x10 -10^{45} .

Decrease of microbial contamination below critical figures was observed on the 5th day of treatment with cucumazyme to 2.3x10 -10^{34}In patients of the second group, where the complex treatment included topical cucumazyme, at the end of treatment 62% of patients were isolated pathogenic or conditionally pathogenic microorganisms at a concentration of $1.2x10^{3}$ in 1 ml of wound fluid.of the secretion. Absence of microbial growth was observed in 38% of the examined patients.

Microbiological investigations in SDS in group II patients during treatment.

Patient group	Microbial contamination of 1g of tissue.			
	Twenty-four hours			
	1	3	5	9
Cucumazyme	5.2x10 -9 1011	3.1x10 -4 105*	2.3x10 -3 104*	1,2x103*

Note: *- p<0.05.

Microbiological investigations in SDS in group II patients at the end of treatment.

Patient groups	Microbial growth %	Microbial contamination	No micro-robotic growth %
Cucumazyme	62%	1,2x103	38%

Immunological studies showed a significant increase in relative T lymphocyte counts to 52.7 ± 1.8% and T suppressors to 19.8±1.7% (p<0.001).

Immunity indices of group II patients at the end of treatment.

Indicators	On admission	At the end of the treatment
T-lymphocytes %	1000,6±37,7 46,7±1,7	1122,5±56,7 52,7±1,8*
T-helpers %	673,7±34,8 27,8±2	705±33,3 28,3±1,3
T-suppressors %	327,3±17 15,3±1,3	417,5±56,7 19,±1,7*
B-lymphocytes %	383,3±41,7 25,2±1,2	442,7±28,3 21,2±1,8
0-lymphocytes %	425,8±52,1 30,2±2	364,7±32,7 21,8±2,3*
Phagocytic count %	46,3±1,5	51,2±3,2
Ig A g/l	1,1±0,04	1,1±0,01
Ig M g/l	3,4±0,3	1,5±0,2**
Ig G g/l	13,7±0,4	11,6±0,3**
Lysozyme mg%	1,5±0,2	1,75±0,1

Note: *- p<0.05; **- p<0.001 in relation to baseline values.

There was a significant decrease in the absolute content of B lymphocytes to 442.7 ± 28.3cl/μl and in the relative index of 0 lymphocytes to 21.8 ± 2.3% (p<0.05). In the study of humoral immunity there was a tendency for the content of immunoglobulins to approach the norm. The content of lysozyme in serum levels at the end of treatment remained low at 1.75 ± 0.1 (p>0.001) compared to baseline.Morphological studies of biopsy specimens and smear-prints taken from purulent-necrotic wounds of the lower limbs during treatment with cucumazyme showed some positive dynamics, consisting in a decrease in the number of neutrophils in the field of vision, in histological preparations there was a decrease in leukocytic-plasmacytic infiltration of tissues.Thus, local application of cucumazyme led to the delimitation of purulent-necrotic process, which contributed to obtaining excellent and good results in 90.4% of cases. In 47 patients opened purulent foci, necrectomies and disarticulation of fingers with removal of tendons and metatarsal bones were independent operations and not a stage of preparation for high amputation. Amputations at the thigh level were performed in 8 patients (9.8%). The lethal outcome was observed in 1 case. Duration of treatment of patients of group II was equal to 16.6±1.5 days.There was a significant decrease in the absolute content of B lymphocytes to 442.7 ± 28.3cl/μl and in the relative index of 0 lymphocytes to 21.8 ± 2.3% (p<0.05). In the study of humoral immunity there was a tendency for the content of immunoglobulins to approach the norm. The content of lysozyme in blood serum at the end of treatment remained low - 1.75 ± 0.1 (p>0.001) compared to the initial data.

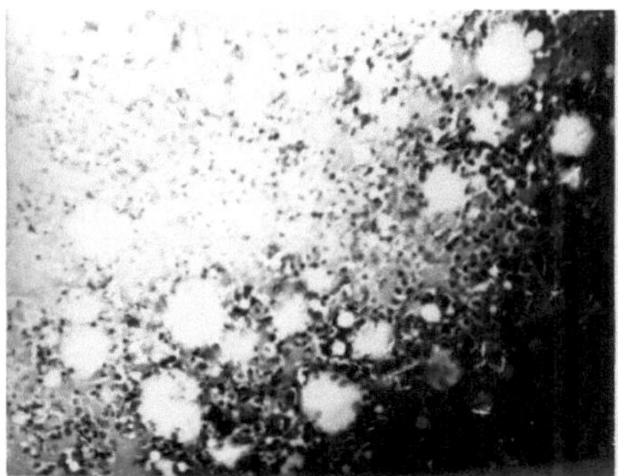

Figure 12: Some reduction of inflammatory elements with cucumazyme treatment. Smear impression. Light microscopy. Haematoxylin-eosin staining. Eq.x160.

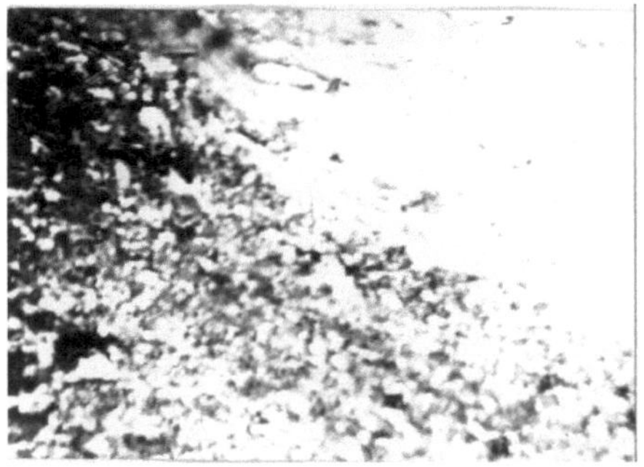

Figure 13: Decrease in leucocytic infiltration with cucumazyme treatment. Light microscopy. Haematoxylin-eosin staining. Eq.x160.

Results of complex treatment of purulent-necrotic complications of the lower limbs with the use of cucumazyme and USC.

Combined application of cucumazyme and ultrasound was performed in 95 patients, among whom neuropathic form was found in 44, osteoarthropathic in 24, ischaemic in 6 and mixed in 21 patients. Improvement of the general condition on the background of the conducted complex therapy with local application of cucumazyme with USC was observed in 94% of patients starting from 2-3 sessions of treatment. Reduction of dull, diffuse pain in the extremities was observed after the 2nd session of USC with cucumazyme. Paresthesias characterised by tingling sensation, "humming", "burning" after treatment disappeared after 3 sessions of treatment. Sensations of numbness of distal limbs were not observed in 89% of patients after 3-4 sessions. Painful cramps in the extremities on the background of ultrasound treatment with cucumazyme were eliminated in 84% of patients after 4-5 sessions.

Results of examination of patients of group III.

Clinical signs	Result
Improvement of general condition	94%
Disappearance of the burning sensation	92%
Reduction in diffuse pain	82%
Disappearance of numbness in the limb	89%
Disappearance of painful cramps in the limb	84%
Distance extension passable without pain	48%

After 2-3 sessions of USC with cucumazyme during dressings or surgeries, significant bleeding of soft tissues was observed, which indirectly indicated good microcirculation of the distal parts of the limb. On laboratory and instrumental investigations, there was a significant increase in LPI to 1.01±0.019, RI to 0.58±0.01 and Max A to 20.1±0.25 cm/s ($p<0.05$).

Indicators of instrumental and laboratory investigations at the of group III patients.

Indicators	Before treatment	After treatment
LPI	0,92±0,01	1,01±0,018*
RI	0,57±0,01	0,58±0,01
MaxA cm/s	18,1±0,4	20,1±0,25*
PTI%	99,4±2,9	82,9±1,6*
Fibrinogen g/l	6,7±0,36	4,78±0,25*
Blood glucose	7,5±0,5	7,8±0,5

Note: *-p<0.05 compared to before treatment.

Treatment indicators in the third group of patients.

Indicators	0	I-II	III	IV	V	Total
Total number of patients	6	20	29	31	9	95 (100%)
Operated on	-	4	25	24	9	62 (65,2%)
Cf. bed day	-	14	22	19	34,5	27±
P/o complications	-	-	-	-	1	1(1,61%)
Lethality	-	-	-	-	1	1 (1,61%)-
Unoperated	6	16	4	7	-	33 (34,8%)
Cf. bed day	12	17,1±1,8	23,7	18,1	-	17,2±
Lethality	-	-	-	-	-	-

16 patients with I-II stage of SDS underwent conservative therapeutic measures. Superficial and deep trophic ulcers were found in 20 patients of the third group. Local ultrasound with cucumazyme was performed during dressings. The ulcer defect was filled with 50 PE of cucumazyme and ultrasound was applied at a distance of 0.5 cm from the ulcer surface. Edema, hyperaemia of the skin disappeared on average after 5 sessions. The dressing was finished by inserting a turunda moistened with cucumazyme solution. On the 2-3 day the surface of trophic ulcers was cleaned from the purulent fibrinous plaque.Appearance of tender granulation tissue was observed on the 5th day of treatment. Complete healing of ulcers was observed on the 11th-12th day in 16 patients (80%). Taking into account the destructive form of osteoarthropathic form of SDS, 3 patients underwent disarticulation of the affected toe with removal of the metatarsal bone head. The average treatment period was 17.1±1.8 days. In 4 patients with stage III SDS it was possible to completely stop the signs of inflammation, suspend the purulent-inflammatory process. Of 29 patients with Stage III 25 patients underwent surgical interventions. 13 patients (with neuropathy-7, osteoarthropathy-1, mixed form-5) underwent phlegmon dissection. In 3 cases (with neuropathy-2, mixed form-1), taking into account the involvement of II-III fingers in the purulent-necrotic process, the operation was performed. was combined with amputation of the toes. In 2 patients with osteomyelitic phlegmon (destructive form of osteoarthropathy), sequestrectomy or removal of the affected metatarsal bones was performed during amputation of the toe and opening of the phlegmon.

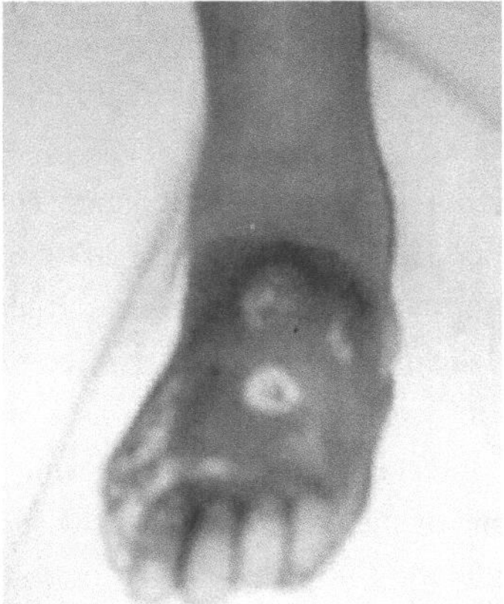

Figure 14: View of a foot with stage III lesions before treatment.

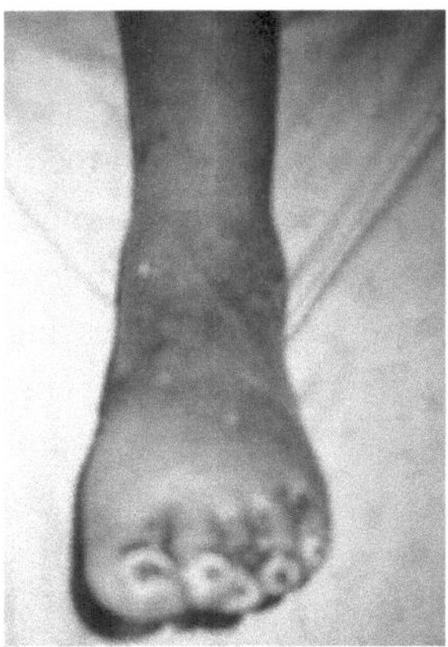

Figure 15. View of the same foot after treatment with USC and cucumazyme.

The final stage of surgery in all cases was ultrasonic treatment of the wound surface with cucumazyme solutions for 10 minutes and insertion of tissues soaked in cucumazyme solution. The obligatory condition was limb unloading, which was performed by bed rest. After the operation 6 patients with diabetic osteoarthropathy received a removable plaster cast for 2 weeks. Daily dressings were continued with CPC with cucumazyme. Increased wound separation was observed for 2-3 days. On the average the wound clearing from purulent-necrotic masses was observed on 9.2±0.3 days. By 10,9±0,3 day granulation tissue appeared on the wound surface. In order to accelerate the healing time by this period 5 patients had rare sutures put on the wound. Wound healing occurred on 16.1 ± 0.7 days. A total of 147 sessions of USC or 5 sessions per one patient were performed. The average treatment period of the operated patients with stage III was 22±1.5 days. In stage IV with the presence of wet necrotic process, 7 patients underwent USC and cucumazyme applications. Good results were obtained in 7 cases (22.3%) after 6-7 sessions of ultrasonic treatment and local therapy with cucumazyme. Reduction of foot oedema, hyperaemia was noted on the 3-4 day. Complete rejection of necrotic tissues was observed on the 7th day in 3 patients. In other cases wet necrosis turned into a dry form. No operative interventions were performed in these patients. The average terms of treatment of patients made 18,1±1,1 days. With stage IV foot lesions, 24 patients underwent surgical interventions. 2 patients with the ischaemic form underwent reconstructive surgery on the vessels of the lower limb in vascular surgery departments after consultation with an angiosurgeon. 14 patients underwent finger amputations with removal of tendon-synovial sheaths.

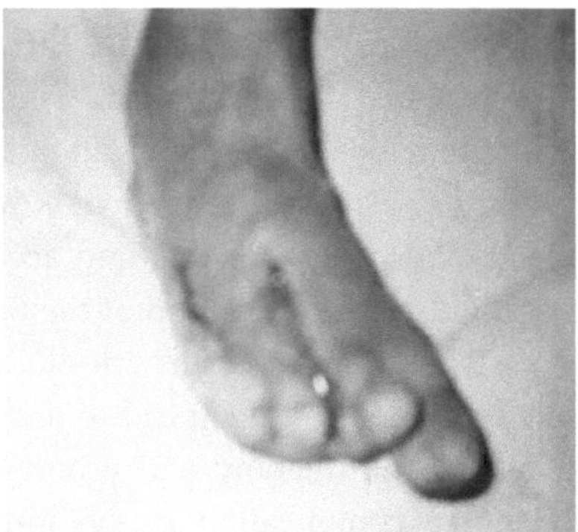

Figure 16. Amputation of the third finger with tendon removal.

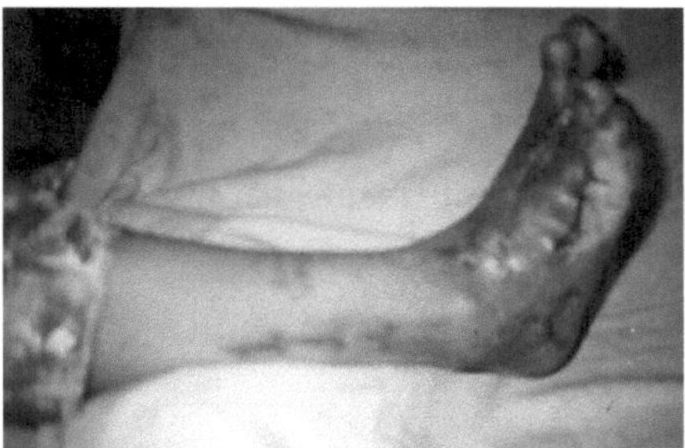

Fig. 17: Removal of the tendon with an incision extended to the lower third of the tibia in the same patient.

In 2 patients, given the involvement of tendons in the purulent-necrotic process, this incision was extended to the lower third of the tibia. The operation was finished by applying converging sutures to the wound. One patient after delimitation of the necrotic process underwent Sharpe's foot amputation. High limb amputations were performed in 3 patients taking into account the progression of purulent-necrotic process to the lower leg and ineffectiveness of the treatment. No postoperative complications were observed. The average time of treatment of patients was 19 days. Special efforts were required in patients with stage V of limb damage by purulent-necrotic processes. In 7 patients on the background of ultrasound and local application of cucumazyme it was possible to stop purulent-necrotic process, localise the purulent process. In 2 patients the purulent centre was opened with amputation of the toes. In 6 cases staged necrectomies were performed. Dressings were supplemented with USC with cucumazyme, wounds were loosely tamponated with gauze turundas moistened with cucumazyme solution. Clearing of wounds from purulent-necrotic layer was observed at 9.2 ± 0.3 days. Necrotic tissues were easily removed. By 8 days tender granulation tissue appeared in the wound. The wounds bled easily, indicating improved blood circulation. After granulation appeared, we switched to ointment dressings. Mostly water-soluble ointments based on polyethylene oxide were used. 2 patients underwent skin grafting according to Tirsch. The skin flap in the anterior surface of the upper third of the thigh was taken using a Tirsch knife. The first dressing was made on the 5th-6th day. In other cases the wounds healed by secondary tension. 1 patient had to undergo thigh amputation due to the lack of effect from the therapy and progression of the purulent-necrotic process. Postoperative complication in the form of infiltrate of the femoral stump wound was observed in 1 patient. There were no lethal outcomes. Microbiological studies in the third group of patients showed that the combined application of cucumazyme and UPC contributed to a significant decrease in microbial contamination after 3 sessions of treatment to 3.5x10 -10[34]

Microbiological studies in purulent-necrotic complications of lower extremities in diabetic patients at the end of treatment.

Patient group	Microbial contamination of 1g of tissue.			
	Twenty-four hours			
	1	3	5	9
Cucumazyme+PCM	4.9x10 -8 1010	3.5x10 -3 104	1.9x10 -2 103	1.2x10 -2 103

Significant reduction of microbial contamination ($1.2x10^2$-10^3) below critical figures was observed when ultrasound cavitation of wounds was connected in 48% of patients at the end of treatment. In this group the absence of microbial growth was observed in 52% of the examined patients.

Microbiological studies in group III patients at the end of treatment.

Patient group	Microbial growth %	Microbial contamination	Absence of micro- %
Cucumazyme+PCM	48%	1.2x102 -103	52%

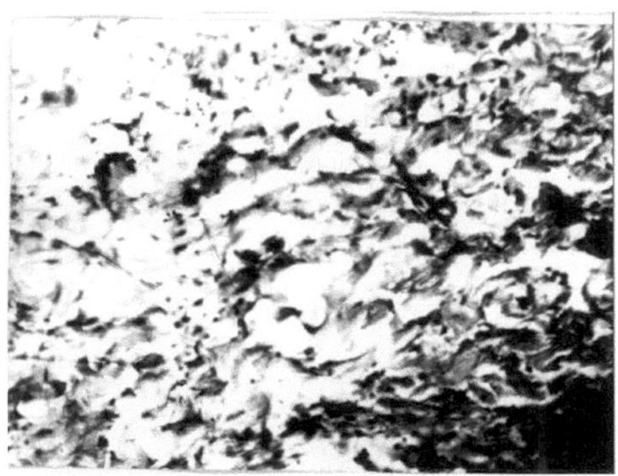

Fig. 18. Noticeable reduction of inflammatory process, development of fibroplastic processes with combined application of cucumazyme and USC. Light microscopy. Haematoxylin-eosin staining. Eq.x160.

In immunological studies, there was a significant increase in both absolute and relative content of the total pool of T-lymphocytes to 1153.3±41.7 and 55.5±1.8, T-helpers to 28.5±3, and T-suppressors to 370.3±26.3%, respectively. There was also a non-significant increase in B and a decrease in 0-lymphocytes. At the end of treatment there was an increase in phagocytic number up to 52,7±1,7% ($p>0,05$).Combined treatment of purulent-necrotic wounds of the lower limbs with local application of cucumazyme and ultrasound results in a marked reduction of inflammatory processes, along with the activation of regenerative-proliferative mechanisms, which is confirmed by a decrease in the number of necrotic masses, the appearance of immature fibroblasts, plasma cells in the wound area.

Immunity indices of group III patients with purulent-necrotic complications of lower limbs in diabetes mellitus at the end of treatment.

Indicators	On admission	At the end of the treatment
T-lymphocytes %	1025,3±59,7 49,5±1,7	1153,3±41,7 55,5±1,8*
T-helper cells %	741±47,8 26,7±4,2	766,3±34,7 28,5±3*
T-suppressors %	284,2±33,3 12,8±1,6	370,3±26,3* 15,5±1,3
B-lymphocytes %	337,5±48,8 28,8±2,3	577,5±47,5* 27,7±1,8
0-lymphocytes %	244,3±60 21,2±3,3	234,5±56,8 17±3,3
Phagocytic count %	48,7±2	52,7±1,7
Ig A	1,2±0,03	1,3±0,04*
Ig M	3,6±0,3	2±0,2*
Ig G	13,6±0,3	11,9±0,4*
Lysozyme	1,3±0,1	1,7±0,2*

Note: * - $p<0.05$ in relation to baseline values.

In cytological preparations, there are heavy, layers of fibroblasts, fibrin films with single neutrophils, degenerating cells Of the 95 patients in the third group, 62 (65.3%) underwent surgical interventions.

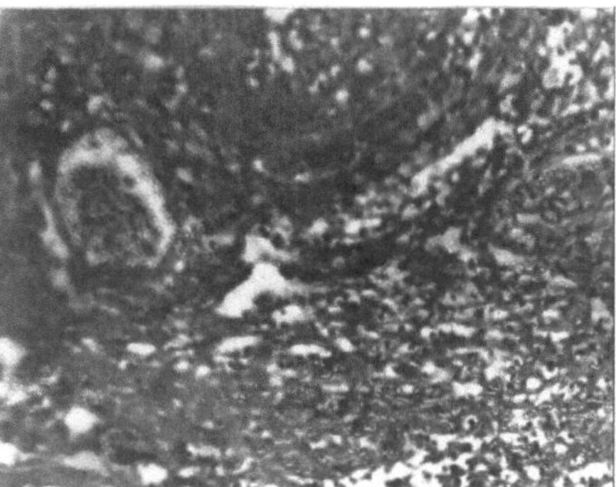

Fig. 19: Appearance of immature fibroblasts, plasma cells with combined application of cucumazyme and USC. Light microscopy. Haematoxylin-eosin staining. Eq.x160.

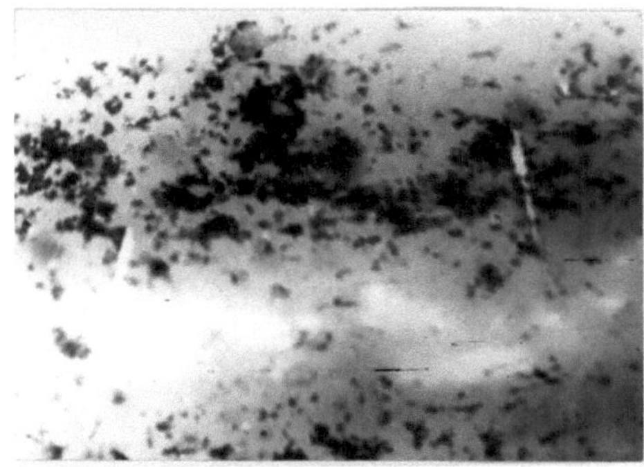

Fig. 20. Heavings, fibroblast strata with single neutrophils in combined application of cucumazyme and USC. Light microscopy. Haematoxylin-eosin staining. Eq.x160.

Results of complex treatment of purulent-necrotic complications of the lower extremities in diabetes mellitus with the inclusion of autotransfusion with UV-irradiated blood, cucumazyme, and CBC.

In this subchapter we present the results of treatment of patients with the inclusion of AUVOC with local application of cucumazyme and USC, we studied the course of different clinical forms under the influence of AUVOC. With neuropathic form there were 36, osteoarthropathic 10, ischaemic 5 and mixed 11 patients. The frequency of AUVOC use was also depended on the form and stage of the patients' general condition. A total of 348 sessions of AUVOC or 5.6 per 1 patient were used. In the presence of purulent-necrotic process the treatment was supplemented with ultrasound treatment with cucumazyme. Otherwise, the complex treatment measures did not differ in comparison with other groups of patients. Blood glucose on admission was 9.2 ± 0.8 mmol/l. 9 patients received sugar-lowering drugs in tablet form. 53 patients were switched to simple insulin from the first days of treatment. The daily dose of insulin was 18-24 units. Reduction of glycaemia level was noted along with improvement of clinical manifestations of neuropathy and ischaemia up to 7.7±0.4 ($p>0.05$). The results of the study in group IV testify to the positive effect of AUFOC on ischaemic and mixed forms of SDS. The pronounced effect was observed in 55 (88,7%) patients, moderate - in 5 (8%). AUVOC had a significant positive effect on the course of the disease. After the 2nd session of AUFOC in 9 patients disappearance of so-called small signs of ischaemia was noted: increased feeling to cold, chilliness, early leg fatigue, cramps, paresthesias in the form of creeping goosebumps, feeling of foot numbness. Since each patient did not necessarily have all the above-mentioned complaints and had an individual symptom-complex, the change of complaints on the background of AUFOC was also individual. In 2 patients with the I degree of ischaemia the most rapid improvement of the condition occurred, they had no complaints at all, and after 4-5 procedures they stopped the treatment on their own. interrupted treatment motivating this complete disappearance of leg discomfort and increased tolerance to physical activity.

Patients after 4-5 sessions of AUFOC noted a decrease or absence of pain syndrome at rest, at night. Tolerance to physical load increased after each session, intermittent claudication appeared after travelling a greater distance. It should be especially noted that after the course of AUFOC in patients with ischaemia the symptom of intermittent claudication was completely absent, which indicates a decrease in the degree of ischaemia. In patients baseline reserve possibilities blood circulation lower extremities were low. This was significantly confirmed by RVG (RI-0.6 ± 0.002) and USDG (Max A 19.5 ± 0.4 cm/s) data, according to which in the lower limbs of the In the limbs, a decrease in volume blood flow was detected. The symptom of intermittent claudication appeared when walking a distance of less than 100-300 metres. By the end of treatment tolerance to load increased 3 times, patients noted normalisation of sleep, improvement of general well-being and mood. No significant effect of treatment was observed in 2 (12.5%) patients. According to RVG and USDG data, peripheral blood flow in the lower extremities significantly improved.

Our studies (RVG and USG data) confirmed the preservation of the main blood flow in the limb in 21 patients, which was the reason to establish the presence of microangiopathy in them. Unfortunately, the prevalence of diffuse microangiopathy is the main factor that leads to ischaemic condition, and in such cases, the conduction of the reconstructive surgeries on the vessels of the lower limb do not give the desired effect.

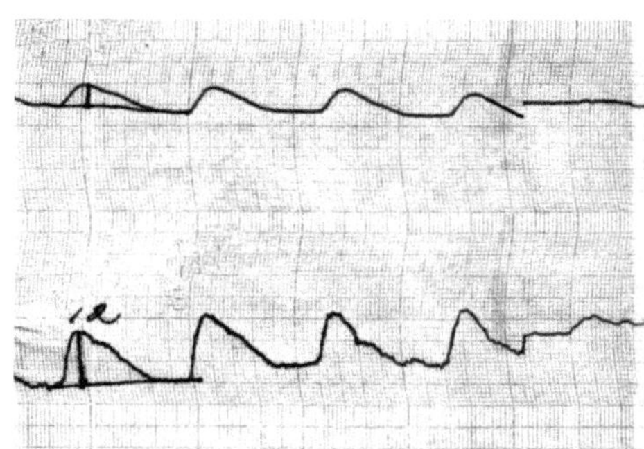

Figure 21: RVG of a patient with ischaemic SDS before treatment.

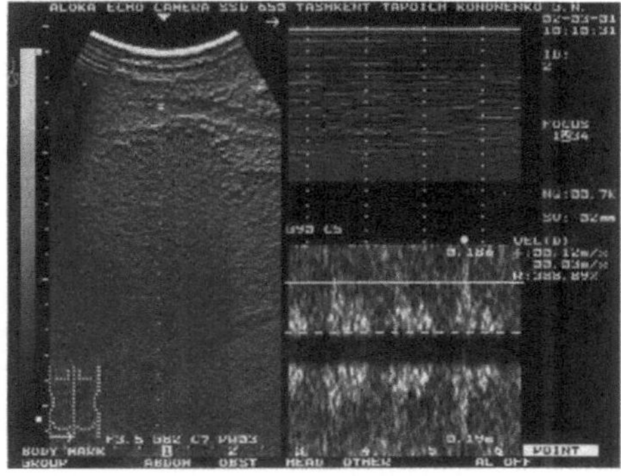

Figure 22: USDG of a patient with grade III ischaemia before treatment.

Out of 62 patients of the fourth group, 41 (66.1%) underwent surgical interventions. All patients in this group underwent AUVOC in combination with ultrasonic treatment and topical application of cucumazyme. The number of AUVOC procedures depended on the clinical form of foot lesions, depth and spread of purulent-necrotic process.

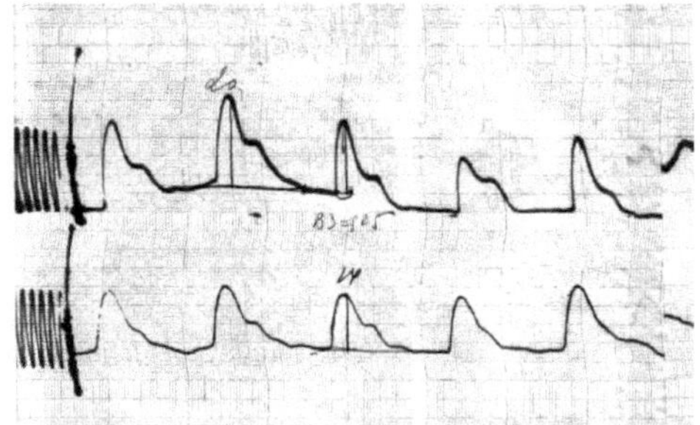

Figure 23: RVG after treatment following AUFOC treatment.

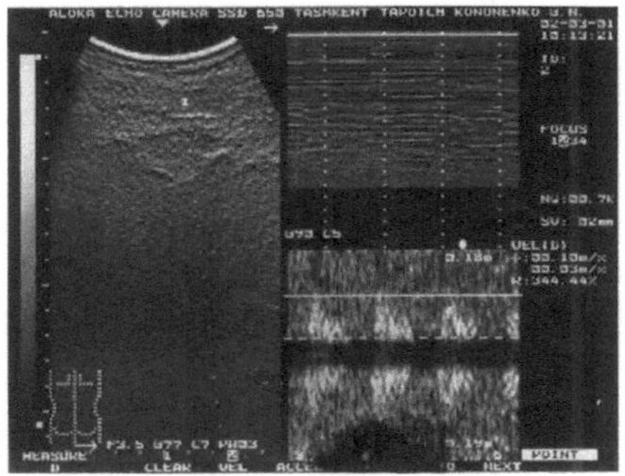

Figure 24. USDG after treatment with AUFOC.

Indicators of instrumental and laboratory studies of patients during combined application of AUFOC to patients with ischaemic and mixed forms of diabetic foot.

Indicators	Before treatment	After treatment
LPI	0,93±0,01	0,99±0,01*
RI	0,56±0,01	0,60±0,002*
MaxA cm/s	17,5±0,5	19,5±0,4*
PTI %	96,8±2,9	81,0±2,9*
Fibrinogen g/l	5,6±0,5	3,9±0,2*
Blood glucose mmol/l	9,2±0,8	7,7±0,4
Glucose in the urine	More than 3 per cent	1%

Note: p<0.05 compared to before treatment.

5 patients with stage 0, when there was no purulent-necrotic process, had 5 sessions of AUVOC. Improvement of the general condition, reduction of pain syndrome in the limb were noted by all 5 patients after 3-4 AUVOC sessions.

Treatment indicators in the fourth group of patients.

Indicators	0	I-II	III	IV	V	Total
Total number of patients	5	14	18	20	5	62 (100%)
Operated on	-	7	14	18	3	42 (67,7%)
Cf. bed day	-	15,4	25	27,1	21	25,7±
Unoperated	5	7	4	2	2	20 (32,3%)
Cf. bed day	13,8	24	19,7	20,6	30	20,8±

In I-II stage of SDS in 7 cases healing of ulcers with formation of a tender scar was observed by 7 days. 7 patients with localisation of deep trophic ulcers on the toes of the foot and pronounced deformation of these toes on the background of destructive osteoarthropathy underwent finger disarticulation. Primary sutures were applied to the wounds after finger disarticulation, which were removed on the 9th-10th day. The wounds healed with primary tension in all cases. In patients with stage III AUVOC was performed from the first day of treatment. Surgical interventions were performed in 14 patients. 5 patients on the next day of admission underwent emptying of the purulent focus with radical necrectomy, necrotically changed tissues were removed. In 3 patients, taking into account the combined lesion of the fingers, amputation of the toes with removal of tendons and synovial sheaths was performed. 8 patients underwent staged necrectomies. Wound ultrasound treatment with antiseptic solutions was performed from the first days. The wounds were loosely tamponated with cucumazyme solution. After 2-3 sessions of AUFOC the patients' general well-being improved. Body temperature normalised, appetite improved, sleep normalised. Blood sugar decreased from 10.23 ± 1.03 to 5.41 ± 0.28 ($p<0.05$). The appearance of granulation in the wound was noted on 11.3 ± 1.9 days of treatment on average. Early secondary sutures were applied to accelerate wound healing. In the presence of large cavities, especially after opening of phlegmon and removal of tendon-synovial sheaths, wound closure was supplemented by inserting drainage tubes into the wound cavity (5 patients). The wound cavity was washed with antiseptic and cucumazyme solutions through the drainage tubes. Complete wound healing was observed on 16.2 ± 2.2 days. The average treatment period of the operated patients was 25.7 ± 1.5 days. In 4 cases active conservative measures with connection of AUFOC, ultrasound treatment and cucumazyme promoted delimitation of purulent-inflammatory process, rejection of necrotic tissues and appearance of granulation. Subsequently, wound dressings were performed with ointment preparations on polyethylene oxide base (levomekol). These patients were discharged from the hospital without surgical intervention. The average time of treatment of unoperated patients was 19.7+1.2 days. In stage IV AUVOC was performed taking into account the clinical forms of foot lesions. On average, 8 and 6 AUVOC sessions were applied per treatment course, respectively. UZK and cucumazyme were applied from the first day of patients' admission to the hospital. In 12 patients by 5 days separation of purulent-necrotic process with transition of wet purulent-necrotic process to dry necrosis was observed. In 3 patients, taking into account mummification of necrotically changed finger, surgical intervention was not performed. 10 patients underwent necrectomy. 2 patients underwent emptying of the purulent centre with subsequent necrectomy. In these cases opening of the purulent centre and necrectomies were the final operation. Amputation and disarticulation of the toes were performed in 11 patients. In 6 cases the operation was supplemented by removal of flexor tendons with synovial sheaths, in 2 cases of them, taking into account destructive osteoarthropathy, the corresponding metatarsal bones were additionally removed. In all cases of toe amputations the operation was completed by primary suturing of the wound, and primary wound healing was noted in all patients. Foot amputations were performed in 2 patients.

Frequency of application of AUFOC, USC and cucumazyme in the fourth group of patients.

Type of treatment	0 n-5	I-II n-14	III n-18	IV n-20	V n-5
CPC total Per 1 patient	-	70 5	109 6,05	152 7,6	42 8,4
Cucumazim total Per 1 patient	-	122 4,02	158 8,7	178 8,9	48 9,6
AUFOC total Per 1 patient	25 5	70 5	98 5,4	122 6,1	33 6,6

In 1 case, all toes of the foot were separated according to Gorangeau with resection of the metatarsal heads (Fig.25). In one case, Sharpe amputation was performed. The average time of treatment of patients with stage IV was 17.1+1.0 days. In 4 cases by 5 days of treatment it was possible to delimit the necrotic process, and on the 7th day the foot oedema completely subsided. Clearance from purulent-necrotic tissues occurred on 8.5+0.4 days (Fig.4.4.7).
2 patients with stage V SDS underwent staged necrectomies. The liquefied necrotic tissues were easily removed. Appearance of granulation tissue was observed on 11.1+0.4 days. Wound healing occurred on 16.3±0.5 days. In 1 case with heel gangrene, the limb was saved without surgical treatment.

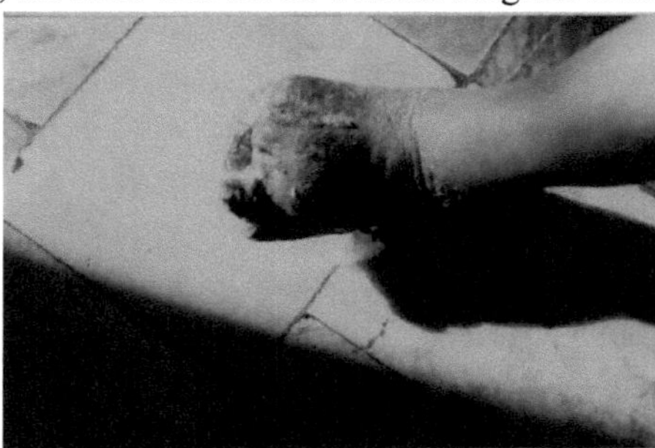

Fig. 25. Horangeau toe separation.

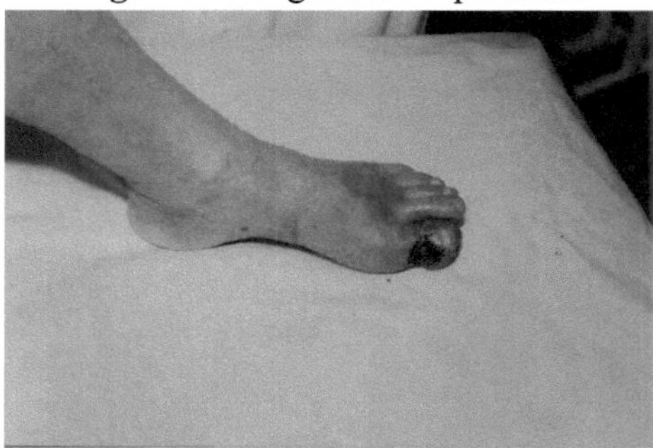

Figure 26: Gangrene of the first toe of the left foot before treatment.

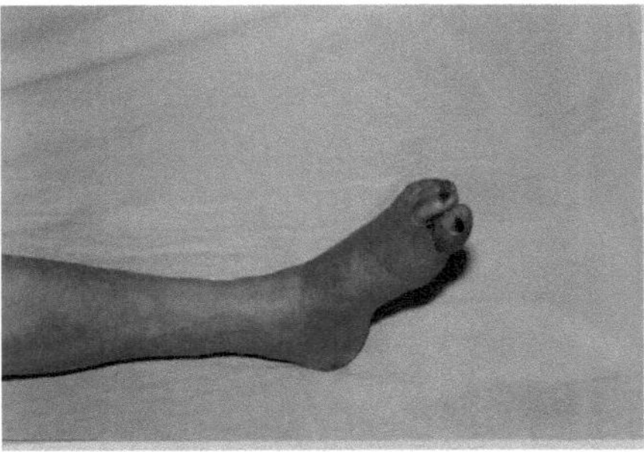

Fig. 27. On the 8th day after treatment with cucumazyme on the background of AUFOC.

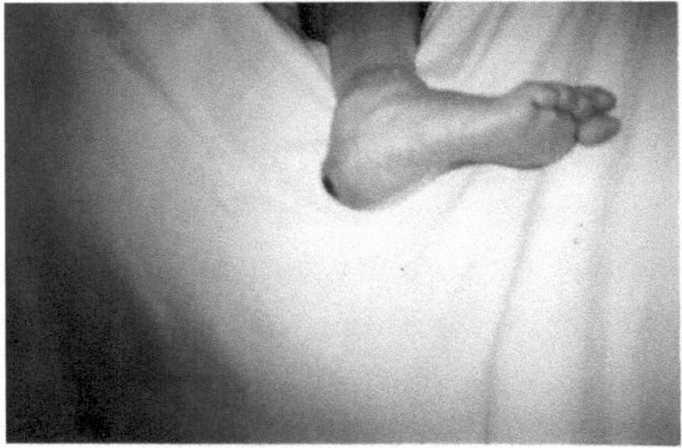

Figure 28. View of a foot with calcaneal gangrene before treatment.

On the 7th day of application of AUFOC, USC and cucumazyme it was possible to stop purulent-necrotic process.

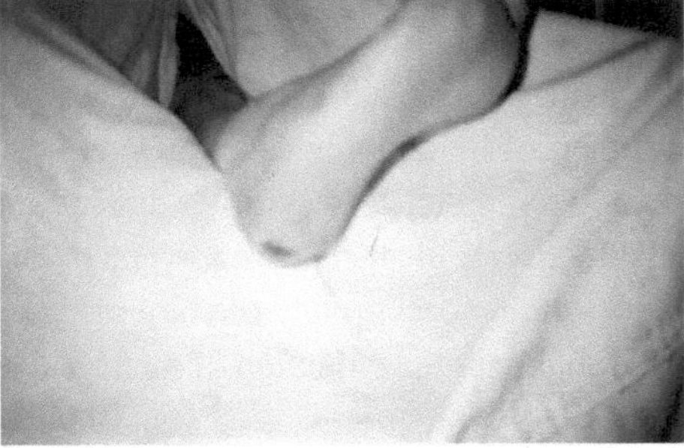

Figure 29. View of the foot on the 7th day of treatment with AUFOC, USC and cucumazyme.

In 1 case, a Pirogov amputation of the tibia was performed (Fig.30.).

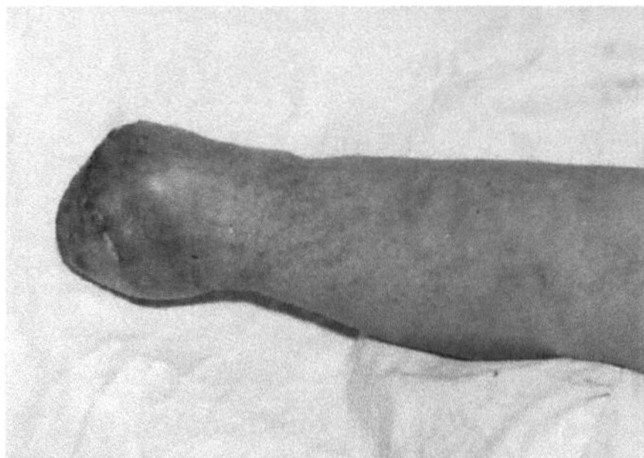

Figure 30. Condition after bone-plastic amputation of the tibia by Pirogov.

2 patients had to undergo hip amputation due to the progression of purulent-necrotic process. Postoperative wound healing in these patients was primary tension. After consultation of a vascular surgeon, reconstructive surgeries were indicated in 2 patients (3.2%), who were subsequently operated on in different vascular surgery departments. Against the background of combined application of AUFOC, ultrasound treatment with cucumazyme there was not only a tendency to normalisation of immunity indices due to the increase in the quantitative content of cellular elements, but also their qualitative improvement, expressed in an unreliable increase in phagocytic number up to 52.3 ± 3.8% ($p>0.05$). At the same time there was also an increase in the content of lysozyme in blood serum up to 1.8±0.2mcg/ml ($p<0.05$). This confirms the opinion that AUVOC, in addition to its bactericidal effect, stimulates the immune system. Probably, the improvement of immunological parameters on the background of AUFOC is to a greater extent connected with its direct bactericidal effect and photomodification of blood cell elements. Improvement of both humoral and cellular immunity indices on the background of combined application of various methods occurred in parallel with the reduction of microbial contamination.

Immunity indices of group IV patients at the end of treatment.

Indicators	On admission	At the end of the treatment
T-lymphocytes	961,8±43,3*	1086,7±56,7
%	46,2±3,8*	52±4
T-helpers	655,3±46,7*	772,8±43,7
%	26,7±2*	31,5±1,7
T-suppressors %	305,8±33,3 16±3,3	310,5±48,3 15,3±1
B-lymphocytes %	391,7±21,7** 25,5±1,7**	512,2±50,5* 28±0,7
0-lymphocytes %	362±29,2** 26,5±4**	324,7±58 20±4,7
Phagocytic count %	46,5±4**	52,3±3,8
Ig A g/l	1,2±0,1**	1,1±0,1
Ig M g/l	3,8±0,3**	1,7±0,1
Ig G g/l	14,1±0,3**	11,3±0,6*
Lysozyme mg%	1,2±0,1**	1,8±0,2**

Note: * - p<0.05. **<0.005 in relation to the initial values

Microbiological investigations in group IV patients during treatment.

Patient groups	Microbial contamination of 1g of tissue.			
	Twenty-four hours			
	1	3	5	9
AUFOC+cucumazyme+PCM	5.3x10 -9 1011	2.9x10 -3 104	1.7x10 -2 103	1.5x10 -1 102

When AUVOC was connected, no microbial growth was noted in the cultures at the end of treatment in 78% of patients.

Microbiological studies of group IV at the end of treatment.

Patient group	Microbial growth %	Microbial contamination of 1 g of tissue	No Microbial growth %
AUFOC+cucumazyme+PCM	22%	1.5x101 -102	78%

Morphological study of biopsy specimens and smears taken from purulent-necrotic wounds of diabetic patients after AUVOC in combination with local application of cucumazyme and ultrasound showed almost complete disappearance of necrotic masses from the field of vision with "cleansing" of the wound surface, a tendency to revascularisation of the damaged tissue was noted. Normalisation of the dermis structure with the growth of connective tissue layers is revealed near the wound zones, although one can see zones of edema of the basal layer of the dermis with hyperplasia of skin appendages. In biopsy specimens taken from this category of patients, it was noted along with the presence of fibroblasts, lymphocytes, plasma cells, which indicate the intensity of regenerative processes (Fig.35.).

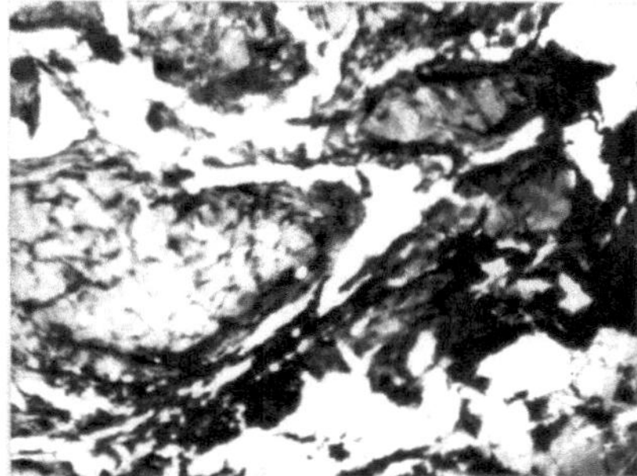

Fig. 31: Disappearance of necrotic masses from the field of vision with combined application of AUVOC, cucumazyme and USC. Light microscopy. Haematoxylin-eosin staining. Eq.x160.

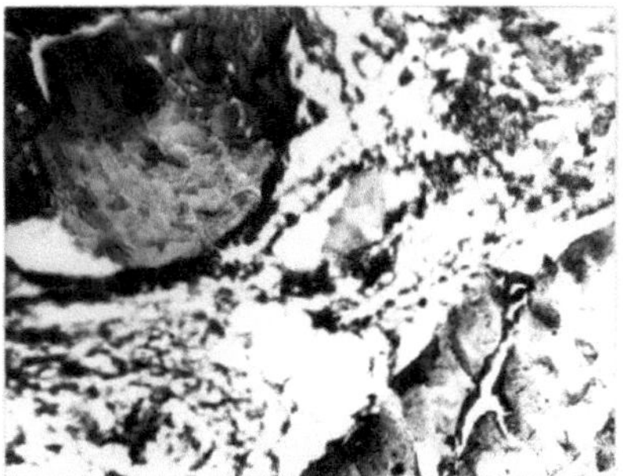

Figure 32. Revascularisation of damaged tissue with combined application of AUVOC, cucumazyme and ultrasound. Light microscopy. Haematoxylin-eosin staining. Eq.x160.

Summarising the results of treatment of patients with purulent-necrotic complications of the lower limbs on the background of DM in the fourth group, where the combination of AUVOC, ultrasound and cucumazyme was included in the complex of treatment measures, we came to the following: excellent and good results were obtained in 93.5% of cases. High limb amputations were performed in 4 patients (6.5%). Fatal outcome was observed in 1 case (1.6%). There was a significant increase in the number of patients with I and II degrees up to 20 (32,3%) and 38 (61,3%) and decrease with III degree of SDS severity up to 4 (6,4%) ($p<0,05$). The positive effect from application of AUFOC in our opinion is carried out by: direct bactericidal, anticoagulant, improving rheological properties of blood and microcirculatory channel actions. The combined use of AUFOC, ultrasound and cucumazyme in the complex treatment of patients with purulent-necrotic complications in the lower extremities against the background of DM with stages IV-V opens up new opportunities for low-traumatic operations on the foot and contributes to the preservation of the supporting function of the foot, which is of great importance. In most cases, conventional necrectomies were radical and were independent operations rather than a stage of preparation of patients for high amputations. Often, the combination of AUVOC with local application of ultrasound and cucumazine lead to suppression of the inflammatory process, contributing to the transition of wet necrotic process to dry form.

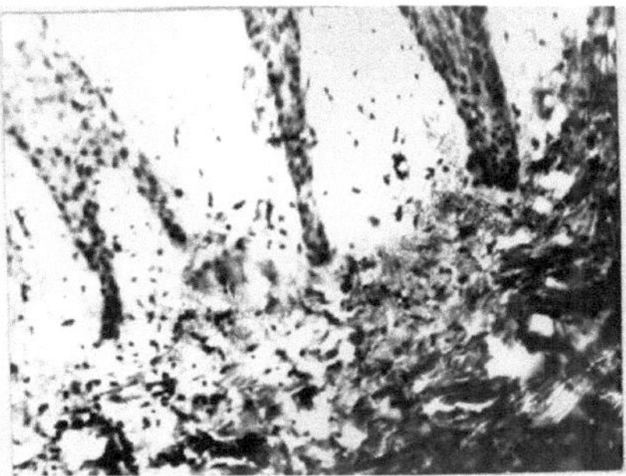

Fig. 33. Expansion of connective tissue layers near purulent-necrotic wound with combined application of AUVOC, cucumazyme and ultrasound. Light microscopy. Haematoxylin-eosin staining. Eq.x160.

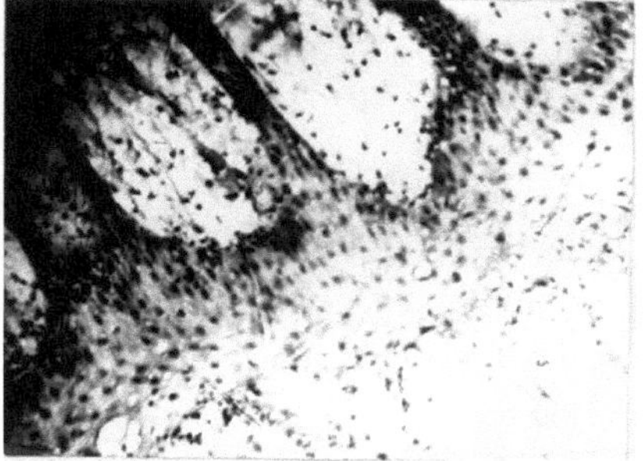

Fig. 34. Moderate oedema of the basal layer of the dermis near the purulent-necrotic wound with combined application of AUVOC, cucumazyme and USC. Light microscopy. Haematoxylin-eosin staining. Eq.x160.

High thigh amputations were performed in 24.1% of patients in the traditional group. The decrease in the frequency of high femoral amputations in the second (9.6%), third (5.3%) and fourth (6.5%) groups of patients cannot be considered only as a result of improved surgical technique or more careful selection of patients, as they have not changed significantly in recent years. The main factor in improving the results of surgical interventions is an optimally developed programme of complex treatment with the inclusion of AUVOC, wound ultrasound and local application of cucumazyme. This is also evidenced by a marked decrease in the number of postoperative complications.

Severity of SDS at the end of treatment.

groups	First Degree,	Grade II,	III degree,	Total
Group I	39 (34,8%)	41 (36,6%)	32 (28,6%)	112 (100%)
Group II	23 (27,7%)	51 (61,5%)*	9 (10,8%)*	83 (100%)
Group III	33 (34,7%)	55 (57,9%)*	7 (7,4%)*	95 (100%)
Group IV	20 (32,3%)*	38 (61,3%)*	4 (6,4%)*	62 (100%)

Note: * - $p<0.05$

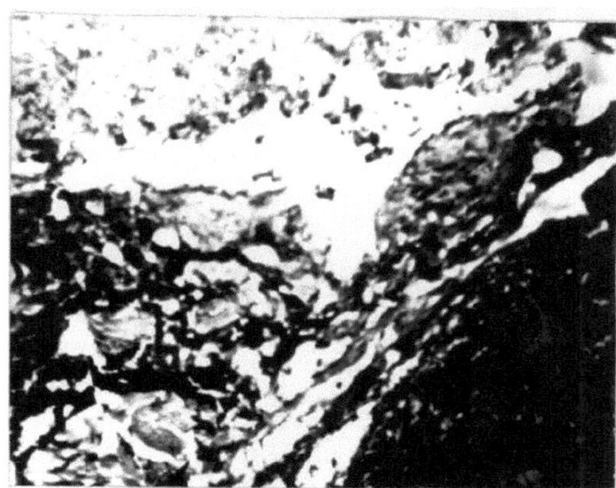

Fig. 35. Thicknesses of fibroblasts, plasma cells, lymphocytes in the area of purulent-necrotic wound with combined application of AUFOC, cucumazyme and USC. Light microscopy. Haematoxylin-eosin staining. Eq.x160.

The treatments we have used (AUVOC, USC and cucumazyme) are accessible, affordable, cost-effective, economical, easy to perform and highly effective, which has been confirmed by our studies. Improvement of clinical signs, favourable course of the wound process in purulent-necrotic complications of the lower extremities in patients with diabetes mellitus on the background of various methods of treatment is due to the reduction of microbial growth and normalisation of immunological parameters. The effectiveness of treatment with the combined use of AUFOC with local the use of cucumazyme and ultrasonic treatment are also confirmed by morphological studies. Application of AUFOC, cucumazyme and USC, judging by morphological data, contributed to a significant reduction of purulent-necrotic process on the one hand, and on the other hand, a tangible positive shift of regenerative-proliferative mechanisms in the damaged tissues of the lower limbs, which correlates with the clinical data.

COMPARATIVE ANALYSIS OF THE EFFECTIVENESS OF THE PROPOSED TREATMENT METHODS AND DEVELOPMENT OF A ALGORITHM OF THERAPEUTIC AND DIAGNOSTIC MEASURES FOR SDS

Comparative analysis of the effectiveness of the proposed methods of treatment of diabetic foot syndrome.

The treatment results were evaluated according to the following criteria, calculated according to the changes in those parameters determining the severity of SDS: -excellent - disappearance of signs of clinical forms of SDS, DM in the stage of compensation, normalisation of laboratory-instrumental parameters, suppression of purulent-necrotic process without surgical intervention; -good - non-critical ischaemia, non-destructive osteoarthropathy, DM in the stage of compensation, normalisation of laboratory and instrumental parameters, delimitation of purulent-necrotic process with subsequent performance of small amputations of the foot with preservation of the supporting function of the limb; -satisfactory - critical ischaemia, destructive osteoarthropathy, DM in the subcompensation stage, significant decrease in immunity indicators compared to the norm, microbial growth above critical figures, presence of detrital and necrotic masses with elements of inflammation, non-bounded purulent-necrotic process with increasing wet gangrene, amputation of the limb at the thigh level with further recovery of the patient; -unsatisfactory - fatal. On the background of traditional therapy improvement of clinical manifestations of SDS forms was observed in 74% of patients. At the same time preservation of expressed clinical manifestations of neuropathy and ischaemia was observed in 58% of patients. Though at 0-I-II stages of SDS the result of traditional therapy was considered excellent, but still in 3 cases we did not observe improvement of clinical manifestations. The terms of clearing, granulation appearance and epithelialisation were delayed. Complete healing of trophic ulcers in the first group was achieved in 11 patients. The suppression and delimitation of purulent-necrotic process on the background of traditional treatment was observed in 80 patients (70.4%), of which 41 patients underwent organ-preserving operations (36.6%). Hip amputations were performed in 27 patients (24,1%). Unsatisfactory results were obtained in 6 cases (5.4%). Postoperative complications were observed in 13 (11.6%) patients, including infiltrate and suppuration of the postoperative wound of the femoral stump (7 patients), continued tissue necrosis (4 cases), and progression of the necrotic process (2 cases). 7 patients died in the postoperative period. The total lethal outcome was 11.6% (13 patients).

Outcomes of conventional treatment depending on the stage of SDS.

Treatment results	0	I-II	III	IV	V	Total
Excellent	10	23	4	2		39(34,8%)
Good			15	25	1	41(36,6%)
Satisfactory			11	5	3	19(17%)
Unsatisfactory			1	8	5	13(11,6%)
Total	10	23	31	39	9	112(100%)

The causes of lethal outcomes were acute myocardial infarction in 4, acute cerebral circulatory failure in 1, and acute multiorgan failure in 2 cases. Among unoperated patients 6 patients died. The main causes of lethal outcomes were growing renal and hepatic insufficiency in 3 patients, acute myocardial infarction in 2 patients and profuse gastrointestinal bleeding in 1 patient. In general, excellent and good results with traditional complex treatment were obtained in 74.1% of cases.

In patients of the second group improvement of the general condition on the background of the conducted therapy (local application of cucumazyme) improvement of the general condition was observed in 94,5% of cases, disappearance of clinical signs of neuropathy and ischaemia was observed in 83-92% of patients.

The suppression and delimitation of purulent-necrotic process succeeded in 74 cases (89.2%), of which 23 patients were treated without surgery. Complete healing of trophic ulcers was observed in 14 (87,5%) out of 16 patients with I-II stages of SDS. 2 patients with I-II stages of SDS after echoosteometric studies performed amputation of the toes with removal of the metatarsal bone heads. A total of 60 patients (72.2%) were operated on. Small amputations of fingers and foot, necrectomies, opening of purulent foci were performed in 51 (61,5%) of them. Application of cucumazyme was effective even at deep destructive processes in the foot. In 23 patients with IV-V stages of SDS it was possible to delimit the purulent-necrotic process, who underwent small amputations of the foot. From 8 patients with V stage in 2 cases it was possible to stop purulent-necrotic process without surgical intervention. Hip amputations were performed in 8 patients (9.6%). Postoperative complications were observed in 1 case. Excellent and good results were obtained in 89.2% of cases. Postoperative lethality was observed in 1 case (1.2%).

The results of treatment in the second group of patients.

Treatment results	0	I-II	III	IV	V	Total
Excellent	7	14	-	-	2	23(27,7%)
Good	-	2	22	23	4	51(61,5%)
Satisfactory	-	-	-	7	1	8(9,6%)
Unsatisfactory	-	-	-	-	1	1(1,2%)
Total	7	16	22	30	8	83(100%)

In the third group, clinical improvement was observed in 94% of patients. 62 patients (65.3%) underwent surgery. 33 patients (34.7%) were treated without surgery. In 16 cases out of 20 patients with I-II stage of SDS combined application of cucumazyme with USC allowed complete healing of trophic ulcers. In 4 cases amputations of the toes were performed, taking into account the changes on echosteometry. In 23 cases (16 patients with I-II stage, 4 with III stage and 7 with IV stage of SDS) the purulent-necrotic process was completely stopped. Organ-preserving operations were performed in 57 patients (60%), who underwent a total of 66 operations.

The results of treatment in the third group of patients.

Treatment results	0	I-II	III	IV	V	Total
Excellent	6	16	4	7	-	33(34,7%)
Good	-	4	25	21	7	55(57,9%)
Satisfactory	-	-	-	3	1	6(6,3%)
Unsatisfactory	-	-	-	-	1	1(1,1%)
Total	6	20	29	31	9	95(100%)

Hip amputations were performed in 6 patients (6.3%). There was 1 lethal outcome (1.1%), which was considered as an unsatisfactory result. It should be noted that in case of deep destructive processes (IV-V stages of SDS) purulent-necrotic process could be stopped in 7 patients with IV stage. Purulent-necrotic process was delimited in 21 patients with IV and 7 patients with V stage of SDS. The combined application of USC and cucumazyme resulted in excellent and good results in 92,6% of cases. The incidence of high limb amputations decreased to 6.3%. Postoperative lethality was observed in 1 case (1.1%). The combined use of AUVOC with local application of cucumazyme and ultrasound resulted in improvement of the general condition in 88.7% of patients. Without surgical interventions 20 patients were treated, of which 15 patients managed to stop purulent-necrotic process. Healing of trophic ulcers was observed in 50% of patients (7 patients). 7 patients with the osteoarthropathic form underwent amputation of fingers with removal of the metatarsal bone heads due to changes in echosteometry. In 9 cases (4 with III, 3 with IV and 2 with V stage of SDS) the necrotic process was completely stopped without surgical intervention. 42 patients (67.7%) were operated on. Small amputations of the foot were performed in 38 patients (61,3%). Hip amputations were performed in only 4 patients (6.5%), of whom 1 patient died (1.6%).

The results of treatment in the fourth group of patients.

Treatment results	0	I-II	III	IV	V	Total
Excellent	5	7	4	2	2	20(32,3%)
Good	-	7	14	16	1	38(61,3%)
Satisfactory	-	-	-	2	1	3(4,8%)
Unsatisfactory	-	-	-	-	1	1(1,6%)
Total	5	14	18	20	5	62

On the background of traditional local therapy the wound clearing from purulent-necrotic layer was observed on 12.1 ± 0.3 days. The appearance of granulation tissue and the beginning of epithelialisation occurred on 14.7±0.3 and 20.3±0.4 days, respectively. Absence of microbial growth in microbiological studies was observed at 9.5±0.5 days. Topical application of the total proteolytic enzyme preparation cucumazyme resulted in cleansing of the wound surface and granulation appearance at 9.7 ± 0.3 ($p<0.05$) and 10.7 ± 0.3 ($p<0.05$) days. Epithelialisation started at 14.7 ± 0.4 days. Cucumazyme having a pronounced proteolytic action contributed to the absence of microbial growth in the wound on 5.0±0.2 days of treatment ($p<0.05$). Reduction of wound cleansing time, granulation appearance and the beginning of the Epithelialisation on the background of combined application of cucumazyme and USC occurred on 9.2 ± 0.3 , 10.9 ± 0.3 and 16.1 ± 0.7 days, respectively ($p<0.05$). The bactericidal effect of USC and cucumazyme contributed to the absence of microbial growth in the wound on 4.5±0.1 days of treatment ($p<0.05$).

Timing of local treatment of patients in different groups.

Timing of treatment	Group I	Group II	Group III	Group IV
Wound cleansing	12,1±0,3	9,7±0,3*	9,2±0,3*	8,5±0,4*
Appearance of granulation	14,7±0,3	10,7±0,3*	10,9±0,3*	11,1±0,4*
Beginning of epithelialisation	20,3±0,4	14,7±0,4*	16,1±0,7*	16,3±0,5*
Duration of treatment	34,4±0,8	21,9±0,4*	23,1±0,5*	24,8±0,5*
Absence microbial growth	9,5±0,5	5,0±0,2*	4,5±0,1*	4,0±0,2*

Note- *-$p<0.05$ compared to the first group.

The combined application of AUVOC, cucumazyme and ultrasound resulted in a shorter period of wound surface cleansing and the appearance of granulation tissue on 3.6 ± 0.4 days, the beginning of epithelialisation on 4.0 ± 0.5 days earlier compared to conventional therapy. The absence of microbial growth was observed on 4.0 ± 0.2 days of treatment.

Algorithm of therapeutic and diagnostic measures in purulent necrotic complications of the lower extremities in patients with diabetes mellitus.

Therapeutic tactics in the development of purulent-necrotic complications is determined not only by the severity of purulent-necrotic manifestations, but also by the form of SDS. This fact makes us follow the diagnostic algorithm, which aims to determine the form of SDS, to identify the localisation and prevalence of the purulent process, as well as possible signs of generalisation of infection. The main goal of surgical treatment of purulent-necrotic manifestations of SDS is to preserve the limb and life of the patient. Since the pathogenesis of neuropathy, osteoarthropathy and ischaemia in SDS is different, then the therapy should be pathogenetic and surgical tactics should differ radically. As literature data have shown, in ischaemic SDS with necrosis in the distal parts of the foot, surgical intervention performed early, even before the appearance of the demarcation zone, almost always leads to the progression of the necrosis zone and is dangerous for the development of wet gangrene. On the contrary, in the neuropathic form of SDS a wide range of surgical interventions is possible. Conservative and surgical measures, which are indicated in the ischaemic form (macroangiopathy), worsen the condition of the neuropathic form, especially with osteoarthropathy, favours the spread of infection, which may eventually lead to high amputation. Based on a comparative study of the results of various treatment methods, we developed an algorithm of therapeutic measures in SDS, taking into account the clinical forms and stage of purulent-necrotic complications of the lower extremities. In doing so, we also took into account the peculiarities of the course of SDS and the results of echosteometric studies.

When a patient with SDS was admitted to the clinic, we determined the depth and prevalence of purulent-necrotic process, i.e. the stage of SDS. If indicated (phlegmon of the plantar spaces of the foot), we performed minor surgical interventions - opening of the abscess, necrectomy. The patient's severe condition due to endotoxaemia due to the progressive purulent-necrotic process was an indication for primary amputation of the limb at the level of the thigh. Clinical-instrumental studies revealed clinical forms of SDS. Clinical neurological studies (vibration, temperature, pain, tactile) were performed to detect the neuropathic form of SDS. Diagnosis of the ischaemic form included examination of the limb and rheovasography, ultrasound Dopplerography and calculation of the ankle-shoulder index. The principle issue in this case is the detection of microangiopathy and macroangiopathy. With the help of clinical examination, foot radiography and echosteometry, the osteoarthropathic form of SDS was diagnosed. It is necessary to determine the presence or absence of destructive process in the bones of the foot by echosteometry. The severity of SDS was determined using the developed scoring scale. The tactics of treatment of purulent-necrotic complications in patients with ischaemic form of SDS is determined by the nature of vascular lesions, the spread of purulent infection and is primarily aimed at reducing the phenomena of critical ischaemia and suppression of purulent process. In ischaemic form of SDS patients were consulted by an angiosurgeon to decide the question of reconstructive surgery on vessels. Most often the distal form of arterial lesions was observed, which in the presence of age-related changes and concomitant diseases limited the possibility of performing reconstructive surgery on the vessels of the lower limb. In the presence of microangiopathy (according to RVG and USG data), vascular therapy was included in the complex treatment, AUVOC, ultrasound treatment with cucumazyme were used. In case of delimitation of purulent-necrotic process in order to preserve the supporting function of the foot, small amputations of the foot were performed. Progression of the purulent-necrotic process, ineffectiveness of reconstructive vascular surgeries, ongoing critical limb ischaemia was an indication for amputation at the thigh level. In case of lesion of the main arteries after consultation of a vascular surgeon, the patients were referred to specialised hospitals for reconstructive vascular surgeries. Reconstructive surgeries were performed in 5 out of 12 patients with critical ischaemia of the lower limb. Due to ineffectiveness of reconstructive vascular interventions, 2 of them underwent forced high limb amputation. In the mixed form of SDS, the complex of therapeutic measures included treatment of neuropathy and ischaemia (alpha-lipoic acid preparations, vascular therapy), AUVOC was applied, local ultrasound treatment with cucumazyme was used. Further tactics depended on the state of necrotic process. When the purulent-necrotic process was isolated, surgical treatment consisted in small amputations of the foot, in case of progression - amputation at the level of the thigh was performed. The treatment of the osteoarthropathic form follows the same rules as for the neuropathic form. Treatment is carried out against the background of lower limb unloading, which is achieved by prescribing bed rest, rest or plaster cast. The choice of therapeutic tactics in the osteoarthropathic form of SDS is necessarily decided taking into account the presence or absence of a destructive process in the bones of the foot. In the absence of destructive process in the

bones of the foot, the complex of therapeutic measures included preventive podiatry treatment (limb unloading, selection of appropriate orthopaedic footwear). If the sound conductivity of the foot bones decreased to 2500m/s and lower on the EOM, i.e. in the presence of destruction of the foot bones, the mandatory stage of surgical interventions was the removal of destructively changed bone areas. In the postoperative period, measures aimed at limb unloading (rest, plaster cast) were continued. Before discharge, patients were recommended to wear appropriate orthopaedic shoes.
Hip amputations should only be performed in the following cases:
- Wet gangrene of the foot with transition to the tibia;
- Critical limb ischaemia with severe pain syndrome when vascular surgery is impossible or conservative therapy is ineffective.
- Destruction of the calcaneus, ankle joint and lower leg bones in diabetic osteoarthropathy.

WHY E

The problem of diabetes mellitus remains one of the most pressing medical and social problems due to its widespread prevalence, tendency to increase in frequency, severity of numerous complications that are difficult to treat. Diabetic foot syndrome is one of the complications of DM, which most often leads to disability and reduced quality of life of patients, occurring in 15% of patients. Lower limb amputations are performed 15 times more often in this group of patients than in the rest of the population. From 50 to 70% of the total number of all amputations of the lower extremities falls on the share of patients with DM [Zemlyanoy A.B. 2003]. The frequency of amputations in patients with diabetes is 17.4-23%, and lethality reaches 9.1%.

The results of studies have shown the necessity of patient management taking into account clinical forms of SDS, depth and spread of purulent necrotic process. Various methods of surgical treatment of neuropathic and ischaemic forms of SDS were proposed, indications and contraindications for their performance were developed.

It is known that neuropathy, ischaemia and infection play a major role in the development of purulent-necrotic processes in the lower extremities. Local therapy of purulent-necrotic processes in the lower extremities in DM with proteolytic enzymes occupies one of the main places in the arsenal of treatment measures for SDS. Preparations of enzymes isolated from microbial and animal material are widely recognised, but preparations of proteolytic enzymes isolated from plants are no less promising. The disadvantage of proteolytic enzymes is their rapid inactivation under the influence of denaturing agents and pH fluctuations. Therefore, proteolytic enzymes have certain requirements: to be resistant, stable to denaturing agents and to retain high activity at different pH parameters of the purulent-necrotic process. In vivo, the biocatalyst is located among a huge set of other macromolecules, so the choice of enzyme mixture is of particular interest. The analysis of information of recent years indicates the possibility and prospectivity of using a complex of proteolytic enzymes of latex of Carica papaya fruits, to which cucumazyme belongs.

Purulent-necrotic processes in the lower extremities in SDS are accompanied by pronounced functional-organic disorders of vital organs and systems. These conditions require the development of such methods of complex therapy, which should be highly effective, accessible, easy to use and have an impact on all pathogenetic links of SDS. In recent years, physical methods of treatment are widely used in the complex of therapeutic measures of purulent-inflammatory diseases. There are reports on the use of autotransfusion of ultraviolet irradiated blood and ultrasound cavitation in the treatment of purulent wounds. However, the results of the effectiveness of these methods in the treatment of SDS remain in the literature are controversial. The influence of AUVOC and ultrasound on the course of clinical forms and stages of SDS is absent.

Recently in the literature there have appeared works, where the results of analyses of the main causes of low efficiency of care for patients with SDS are presented. The main therapeutic and diagnostic errors are considered to be the lack of a differentiated approach to clinical forms of SDS and incorrect assessment of the severity of SDS without taking into account physical, laboratory and instrumental data.

It is necessary to develop an algorithm of therapeutic and diagnostic measures in SDS, allowing timely identification of clinical forms and stages of SDS and to develop gentle methods of complex treatment of destructive forms of diabetic foot, aimed at preserving the support function of the foot.

Further research in this area should be aimed at improving the already known and searching for ways to create new cost-effective, effective and available in use methods of complex treatment for more successful management of the wound process. All the above-mentioned shortcomings were the basis for the present thesis work.

352 patients with purulent-necrotic lesions of the lower limbs against the background of diabetes mellitus were examined. The patients were divided into 4 groups depending on the treatment performed:

Group I - 112 patients who underwent traditional complex treatment including correction of carbohydrate, protein, fat metabolism, rheological properties of blood, improvement of microcirculatory channel, antibiotic therapy, treatment of concomitant pathologies;

II group - 83 patients with purulent-necrotic lesions of the lower limbs against the background of diabetes mellitus, who underwent complex treatment with inclusion of local application of proteolytic domestic enzyme of plant origin cucumazyme;

III group - 95 patients in whom the complex of treatment measures included local application of cucumazyme and USC;

IV group - 62 patients, to whom local application of cucumazyme, ultrasound and AUVOC were included in the complex of treatment measures.

The age of the patients ranged from 17 to 84 years, with a mean age of 62.7 years.

Purulent-necrotic lesions were often found at the age of 45-74 years. Type 1 DM occurred in 23 patients, type 2 DM in 329 patients. Duration of DM - from

6 months to 30 years old. In 18 patients the diagnosis of DM was established on admission to the clinic. Patients in all groups were distributed according to the Wagner classification and WHO. The main contingent of patients came to the clinic later than 3 weeks from the beginning of purulent-necrotic process. The reasons for the patients' late seeking medical help were asymptomatic onset of the disease; absence of pain syndrome; prolonged preservation of skin continuity, which prevents the outflow of the formed pus and necrosis. separation from the pathological focus, self-treatment or inadequate treatment of patients. The degree of DM compensation, clinical form of SDS, prevalence and depth of necrotic process lesion, presence of concomitant pathology determined the therapeutic tactics. The traditional complex of therapeutic measures included correction of glycemia and glucosuria by transferring all patients to short-acting insulin; improvement of blood rheological properties (reopolyglucin, trental, pentoxifylline); correction of coagulopathy under control of coagulogram parameters; detoxification and tonic therapy (haemodez, infusion of electrolytes, protein preparations, plasma and blood); targeted antibiotic therapy taking into account microbiological studies; treatment of concomitant pathologies. It should be noted that in the development of therapeutic measures we considered necessary the participation of endocrinologist, neurologist, and in the ischaemic form we necessarily consulted patients with a vascular surgeon to address the issue of reconstructive surgery on the vessels of the lower extremities.

In local treatment of wounds we used for the first time a total proteolytic enzyme of plant origin - cucumazyme, obtained by the staff of the Institute of Chemistry of Plant Substances of the Academy of Sciences of the Republic of Uzbekistan from the melon tree Carica Papaya and tested with our participation. Cucumazyme was applied topically in a dose of 10mg. (50 proteolytic units). The drug was dissolved in 10ml of 0.5% novocaine solution before use. After opening of the purulent centre, the wounds were loosely filled with a turunda soaked in cucumazyme solution. Dressings were made daily until complete clearing of the wound from purulent-necrotic masses and granulation appearance. AUVOC was performed with the apparatus "UVOC" equipped with the mercury-quartz lamp "DRT-8". The simplicity of AUVOC and USC, which does not require special technical equipment, allows their use in any medical institution. The ultrasonic treatment was performed with the URSK-8T apparatus from the first day of the purulent centre opening. As an antiseptic preparation we used 0.5-1% solution of dioxidine. Purulent cavities were filled with cucumazyme solution and ultrasound was applied at a distance of 0.5-1 cm from the wound wall. Obstetrical, biochemical, immunological, microbiological, and instrumental studies were performed. To assess the state of blood circulation in the lower limb, tetrapolar rheovasography, ultrasound Dopplerography, and ankle-shoulder index were performed. Bone changes were diagnosed using radiological and echosteometric studies. Additionally, chemical analysis of removed bones and bone tissue fragments was performed. The neurological status of the limb was assessed on the basis of podiatric examination. Our studies have shown that in DM the pathogenetic links of purulent-necrotic complications in the lower extremities are as follows neuropathy, osteoarthropathy and angiopathy. The following clinical forms of the course of diabetic foot were found: neuropathy in 52.6%, osteoarthropathy in 17.6%, ischaemic in 6.8% and mixed in 23%, which corresponds to the literature data. At the same time it should be noted that the diagnosis of neuropathic and ischaemic forms of SDS is well developed. Unfortunately, in the literature there is no unified standard of diagnostic measures in osteoarthropathic form of SDS, which leads to contradictory results. To improve the diagnosis of DOAP, we used ultrasound osteometry and chemical analysis of removed bone structures in addition to radiological studies. Our studies have shown that early in the development of SDS the bones of the foot undergo structural changes, which is expressed in the resorption of calcium salts from the bone tissue, which leads to a loss of bone mass. The results of chemical analysis of bones show that destructive processes in the foot develop in those parts of the bone where there is a loss of trace elements, especially calcium less than 2%. By comparing the results of chemical analysis of bones and EOM and conducting correlation analysis between them, a criterion for EOM equal to 2500 m/s was developed. Decrease of sound conductivity on EOM below 2500 m/s indicated the presence of destructive process in bone tissue. At sound conductivity above 2500m/s the destructive process in the bone was absent. The results of the studies allowed us to distinguish two types of osteoarthropathic form - non-destructive and destructive. The conducted studies confirmed that purulent-necrotic processes in the foot at the osteoarthropathic form are a consequence of the primary lesion of bone structures of the foot. This confirms that the development of trophic ulcers and other purulent-necrotic complications is based on the primary destructive changes in the bones of the foot. The results of echoosteometric studies and chemical analysis of bones with regard to clinical manifestations allowed us to come to the following opinion: without denying the role of tendon-synovial sheaths in the spread of purulent-necrotic process, we found that the destructive changes in bones, which remained unnoticed by eye and at radiological studies, can be a source of delay and spread of necrotic process.

Our results require a revision of treatment tactics in osteoarthropathic form of SDS. Surgical treatment of osteoarthropathic SDS is indicated only in the presence of destructive osteoarthropathy. The indication for amputation of the lower limb at the thigh level in osteoarthropathic form of SDS in our opinion is destruction of the calcaneal bone and ankle joint.

Therapeutic tactics in osteoarthropathic form of SDS, chosen depending on the state of bone structures, helped to reduce the frequency of high amputations to 2.9%, preserve the supporting function of the foot in 97.1% of patients and avoid unnecessary surgical interventions. Based on the results obtained, we proposed an addition to the combined classification of SDS taking into account changes in the bones of the foot, which allows to reflect the etiopathogenesis of the lesion, determine the tactics of treatment, has prognostic significance and is easy to apply. Studies also established, that purulent-necrotic complications in the lower extremities, regardless of the clinical form and stage of diabetic foot, proceed with a pronounced decrease in humoral and cellular immunity. There were observed a significant decrease in absolute and relative numbers T-lymphocytes ($p<0,001$). Phagocytic number in the patients examined by us was in reliably ($p<0.001$) low numbers. On admission of patients in all groups we observed significant changes in the indicators of humoral immunity, which was expressed in a significant ($p<0.001$) increase in the content of Ig G and Ig M. Microbiological studies identified aerobic-anaerobic associations, most often including obligate-anaerobic non-spore-forming bacteria (Peptococcus spp., Peptostreptococcus spp.,

Bacteroides fragilis), facultative-anaerobic (Staph. Epidermidis, Staph. Aureus), aerobic microorganisms (Pseudomonas aeruginosa). Microbial contamination of tissues was 10 -10^{512} microorganisms in 1g of tissue. Recently in the literature there have appeared works, where the results of analyses of the main causes of low efficiency of care for patients with SDS are presented. The main therapeutic and diagnostic errors are considered to be the lack of a differentiated approach to clinical forms of SDS and incorrect assessment of the severity of SDS without taking into account physical, laboratory and instrumental data. This setting served as a prerequisite for the creation of a working scale for objective assessment of the severity of patients with purulent necrotic complications of the lower extremities in diabetes mellitus. In doing so, we took into account 8 parameters that most strongly influence the course and outcome of SDS treatment. When creating this scale, we were based on the results of our own studies and the identified features of the course of SDS. On the basis of clinical (forms, stages of SDS), laboratory and instrumental investigations and anamnestic data 3 gradations were allocated, which were estimated by corresponding points (I - 1, II - 2 and III - 4 points). The results were evaluated on a point scale.

As a result of analysing the values of the total score index, 3 degrees of SDS severity were identified:

I degree, mild - from 8 to 10 points. The purulent-necrotic process proceeded with a tendency to delimitation of the infectious process, the prognosis was considered favourable. Small surgical interventions (necrectomies) were mainly performed.

II degree, of medium severity - from 11 to 16 points. These patients underwent emergency surgical interventions only on strict indications (opened purulent foci, drainage). Basically, the operations were performed after thorough preoperative preparation, which was aimed at correcting the detected changes. All operations performed were organ-preserving (small amputations of fingers and feet).

III degree, severe - more than 17 points. The prognosis in this category of patients was considered unfavourable. Taking into account these features, operations in this group were performed after reducing the degree of severity.

Treatment of infected lesions of the feet was carried out taking into account the form of the lesion, the prevalence of infection, the presence of osteomyelitis of the foot, which dictated the choice of tactics of podiatric or surgical management and the need for systemic antibiotic therapy.

Treatment outcomes were evaluated according to the following criteria:

-excellent - when it was possible to control the inflammatory process without surgical intervention;

-good - when it was possible to delimit the necrotic process and transform it into local dry necrosis with subsequent necrectomy or disarticulation of the fingers with preservation of the supporting function of the limb;

-satisfactory - when it is not possible to stop purulent-necrotic process and on the background of growing wet gangrene amputation of the limb at the level of the middle or upper third of the thigh with further recovery of the patient is performed;

-unsatisfactory - ascending moist gangrene of the limb, with extremely severe condition of the patient, marked intoxication, acute failure of vital organs with subsequent death. Improvement of general condition on the background of the conducted complex therapy was observed in 72% of patients.

In instrumental studies on RVG, there was a non-significant increase in RI from 0.55 ± 0.01 to 0.57 ± 0.01 ($p>0.05$). On USDG, there was also a non-significant decrease in Max A from 17.6 ± 0.5 to 19.45 ± 0.78 cm/s ($p>0.05$). PLI increased from 0.89 ± 0.02 to 0.92 ± 0.3 ($p>0.05$), indicating a slight improvement in

blood supply in the limb. Suppression and delimitation of purulent-necrotic process on the background of traditional treatment was observed in 80 patients (70,4%), of which 41 underwent organ-preserving operations
(36,6%). Hip amputations were performed in 27 patients (23.7%). Unsatisfactory results were obtained in 6 cases (5.4%). Postoperative complications were observed in 13 (11.6%) patients, among which there were infiltrate and suppuration of the postoperative wound of the femoral stump (7 patients), continued tissue necrosis [4 cases], progression of the necrotic process (2 cases). In the postoperative period 7 patients died. The total lethal outcome was 11.6% (13 patients). The causes of lethal outcomes were acute myocardial infarction in 4, acute cerebral circulatory failure in 1, acute multiorgan failure in 2 cases. Among unoperated patients 6 patients died. The main causes of lethal outcomes were growing renal and hepatic failure in 3, acute myocardial infarction in 2, and profuse gastrointestinal failure in 2. intestinal bleeding in 1 patient. In general, excellent and good results with traditional complex treatment were obtained in 74.1% of cases.

In patients of the second group improvement of the general condition on the background of the conducted therapy (local application of cucumazyme) improvement of the general condition was observed in 94.5% of cases, disappearance of clinical signs of neuropathy and ischaemia was observed in 83-92% of patients. There was an increase of LPI up to 1.04 ± 0.02 ($p<0.05$). Rheovasograms at the end of treatment clearly showed an increase in RI up to 0.60±0.002. The suppression and delimitation of purulent-necrotic process succeeded in 74 cases [89.2%], of which 23 patients were treated without surgery. Complete healing of trophic ulcers was observed in 14 (87,5%) out of 16 patients with I-II stages of SDS. 2 patients with I-II stages of SDS after echoosteometric studies performed amputation of the toes with removal of the metatarsal bone heads. A total of 60 patients (72.2%) were operated on. Small amputations of fingers and foot, necrectomies, opening of purulent foci were performed in 51 (61,5%) of them. Application of cucumazyme was effective even at deep destructive processes in the foot. In 23 patients with IV-V stages of SDS it was possible to delimit the purulent-necrotic process, who underwent small amputations of the foot. From 8 patients with V stage in 2 cases it was possible to stop purulent-necrotic process without surgical intervention. Hip amputations were performed in 8 patients (9.6%). Postoperative complications were observed in 1 case. Excellent and good results were obtained in 89.2% of cases. Postoperative lethality was observed in 1 case (1.2%).

In the third group, clinical improvement was observed in 94% of patients. 62 patients (65.3%) underwent surgery. 33 patients (34.7%) were treated without surgery. In 16 cases out of 20 patients with I-II stage of SDS combined application of cucumazyme with USC allowed complete healing of trophic ulcers. In 4 cases amputations of the toes were performed, taking into account the changes on echosteometry. In 23 cases (16 patients with I-II stage, 4 with III stage and 7 with IV stage of SDS) the purulent-necrotic process was completely stopped. Organ-preserving operations were performed in 57 patients (60%), who underwent a total of 66 operations. Hip amputations were performed in 5 patients (5.3%) with 1 lethal outcome, which was regarded as an unsatisfactory result. It should be noted that at deep destructive processes (IV-V stages of SDS) purulent-necrotic process could be stopped in 7 patients with IV stage. Purulent-necrotic process was delimited in 21 patients with IV and 7 patients with V stages of SDS. The combined application of USC and cucumazyme resulted in excellent and good results in 94,7% of cases. The incidence of high limb amputations decreased to 5.3%. Postoperative lethality was observed in 1 case (1.1%). The combined use of AUVOC with local application of cucumazyme and ultrasound resulted in improvement of the general condition in 88.7% of patients. Without surgical interventions 20 patients were treated, of which 15 patients managed to relieve the pain purulent-necrotic process. Healing of trophic ulcers was observed in 50% of patients (7 patients). 7 patients with the osteoarthropathic form underwent finger amputation with removal of the metatarsal bone heads due to changes in echosteometry. In 9 cases (4 with III, 3 with IV and 2 with V stage of SDS) the necrotic process was completely stopped without surgical intervention. 42 patients (67.7%) were operated on. Small amputations of the foot were performed in 38 patients (61,3%). Hip amputations were performed in only 4 patients (6.5%), of whom 1 patient was fatal (1.6%).

On the background of traditional local therapy the wound clearing from purulent-necrotic layer was observed on 12.1 ± 0.25 days. The appearance of granulation tissue and the beginning of epithelialisation occurred on 14.7±0.3 and 20.3±0.4 days, respectively. Absence of microbial growth in microbiological studies was observed on 9.5 ± 0.5 days. At traditional methods of treatment of purulent-necrotic wounds of diabetic patients in cytological preparations the presence of neutrophils, macrophages, detritus masses was noted, in histological sections necrotic tissue among elements of skin and subcutaneous tissue was also revealed. Local application of the total proteolytic enzyme preparation cucumazyme resulted in cleansing of the wound surface and granulation appearance at 9.7±0.3 ($p<0.05$) and 10.7±0.3 ($p<0.05$) days. The beginning of epithelialisation occurred at 14.7 ± 0.4 days. Cucumazyme having a pronounced proteolytic action contributed to the absence of microbial growth in the wound on 5.0 ± 0.2 days of treatment ($p<0.05$). Morphological studies of biopsy specimens and smears taken from purulent-necrotic wounds of the lower limbs during treatment with cucumazyme showed some positive dynamics, consisting in a decrease in the number of neutrophils in the field of vision, in histological preparations there was a decrease in leukocytic-plasmacytic infiltration of tissues. The best results were obtained with combined application of cucumazyme and ultrasound treatment. Reduction of wound cleansing time, granulation appearance and the beginning of epithelialisation on the background of combined application of cucumazyme with USC occurred on 9.2 ± 0.3 , 10.9 ± 0.3 and 16.0 ± 0.7 days respectively ($p<0.05$). The bactericidal effect of UPC and cucumazyme contributed to the absence of microbial growth in the wound on 4.5 ± 0.1 days of treatment ($p<0.05$). Combined treatment of purulent-necrotic wounds of the lower limbs with local application of cucumazyme and USC leads to a marked reduction of inflammatory processes, along with the activation of regenerative-proliferative mechanisms, which is confirmed by a decrease in the number of necrotic masses, the appearance of immature fibroblasts, plasma cells in the wound area.

The use of AUFOC with local application of cucumazyme with ultrasound, judging by morphological data, contributed to a significant reduction of purulent-necrotic changes in the tissues on the one hand, on the other hand, a tangible positive shift of regenerative-proliferative mechanisms in the damaged tissues of the lower limbs. Combined application of AUFOC, cucumazyme with ultrasound resulted in reduction of time of wound surface cleansing and appearance of granulation tissue by 3,6±0,4 and the beginning of epithelialisation by 4,0±0,5 days earlier in comparison with traditional therapy. Absence of microbial growth was observed on 4.0±0.2 days of treatment. Improvement of clinical signs, favourable wound course process in purulent-necrotic complications of the lower extremities in patients with diabetes mellitus against the background of various methods of treatment was due to the reduction of microbial growth and normalisation of immunological indicators. Against the background of AUFOC application there was not only a tendency to normalisation of immunity indices due to increase of quantitative content of cellular elements, but also their qualitative improvement expressed in a reliable increase of phagocytic number up to 60,88±1,79% ($p<0,05$). The effectiveness of treatment with combined use of AUVOC with local application of cucumazyme and ultrasound was also confirmed by morphological studies. Morphological study of biopsy specimens and smears taken from purulent-necrotic wounds of diabetic patients after AUVOC in combination with local application of cucumazyme and ultrasound showed almost complete disappearance of necrotic masses from the field of vision with "cleansing" of the wound surface, a tendency to revascularisation of the damaged tissue was noted. In the vicinity of wound zones normalisation of the derma structure with growth of connective tissue layers is revealed, although one can see zones of edema of the basal layer of derma with hyperplasia of skin appendages. In biopsy specimens taken from this category of patients, along with the presence of fibroblasts, lymphocytes, plasma cells, which testify to the intensity of regenerative processes. The combined use of AUVOC, ultrasound and cucumazyme in the complex treatment of patients with purulent-necrotic complications in the lower extremities on the background of DM opens new opportunities for low-traumatic operations on the foot and contributed to the preservation of the foot support function, which is of great importance. In most cases, conventional necrectomies were radical in nature and were independent operations, rather than a stage of preparation of patients for high amputations. Often, the combination of AUVOC with local application of USC and cucumazyme led to the control of the inflammatory process, contributing to the transition of the wet necrotic process to the dry form. Subsequently, the mummified fingers fell off by themselves, not requiring surgical interventions.Based on the results of the study, we developed an algorithm of therapeutic measures in SDS. When a patient with SDS was admitted to the clinic, we determined the depth and prevalence of purulent-necrotic process, i.e. the stage of SDS. If indicated (phlegmon of the plantar spaces of the foot), we performed minor surgical interventions - opening of the abscess, necrectomy. The patient's severe condition due to endotoxaemia due to the progressive purulent-necrotic process was an indication for primary amputation of the limb at the level of the thigh. Clinical and instrumental investigations (neurological examinations, radiography of the foot, determination of pulsation on the arteries of the lower limb) revealed clinical forms of SDS. The choice of therapeutic tactics in osteoarthropathic form of SDS is necessarily decided taking into account the presence or absence of destructive process in the bones of the foot, which is determined by echosteometry. In the absence of destructive process in the bones of the foot, the complex of therapeutic measures included preventive podiatry treatment (limb unloading, selection of appropriate orthopaedic footwear). In the presence of destruction of the bones of the foot, the mandatory stage of surgical interventions was the removal of destructively changed bone areas. In the postoperative period, measures to relieve the limb (rest, plaster cast) are continued. In ischaemic form, the tactics of SDS treatment was determined by the nature of vascular lesions, the spread of purulent infection and was primarily aimed at reducing the phenomena of critical ischaemia and suppression of purulent process. In the presence of microangiopathy (according to RVG and USDG data) the complex treatment included vascular therapy, AUVOC, USC with cucumazyme. In case of lesions of the main arteries after consultation of a vascular surgeon, patients were referred to specialised hospitals for reconstructive operations on vessels. In neuropathic and mixed forms of SDS, the treatment complex included treatment of neuropathy and ischaemia (alpha-lipoic acid preparations, vascular therapy), AUVOC was applied, ultrasound treatment with cucumazyme was applied locally. The scope of surgical treatment depended on the severity of SDS. Small amputations of the foot were performed when the purulent-necrotic process was isolated (11-16 points). Progression of the purulent-necrotic process, ongoing critical limb ischaemia (more than 17 points) was an indication for amputation at the thigh level. Thus, the efforts of surgeons in the management of patients with SDS should be aimed at timely diagnosis of the clinical form of SDS, determination of the depth of the lesion of the foot tissues for the choice of adequate complex treatment to preserve the affected limb.

REFERENCE LIST

1. Avdeeva T.V., Varshavsky I.M., Shabanov N.Y., Boklin A.A. Analysis of the results of surgical treatment of diabetic foot. //Problems of endocrinology. - 1999. -№6. -c.13-18.
2. Agzamkhodjaev S.M., Inogamov Y.V., Muradov D.S. Treatment of wet gangrene of the foot in patients with diabetes //Conference of surgeons, endocrinologists and intensive care specialists. -Ташкент.-1996.-c.3-10.
3. Adamyan A.A., Dobysh S.V., Glyantsev S.P. et al. Treatment of purulent wounds with gelevin and biologically active draining sorbents. //Surgery. -1998. -№ 3. -c.28-30.
4. Akbarov Z.S., Rakhimova G.N., Mukhamedova F.A., Akbarov A.Z. Diabetic neuropathy. -Tashkent, 2001, p. 48.
5. Akbarov Z.S., Rakhimova G.N., Ismailov S.N. va boshk. Amaliy diabetologiya zhadvallarda. -Toshkent, 2007, b. 90.
6. Algorithms of specialised medical care for patients with diabetes mellitus. Edited by I.I. Dedov and M.V. Shestakova -Moscow. -2006. -C. 255.
7. Ametov AS, Doskina EV, Mashenko EA Evaluation of the effectiveness of bivasol in the treatment of postmenopausal osteoporosis in type II diabetes mellitus. //Problems of endocrinology. - 2008. -№6. - pp. 8-12.
8. Antonenko I.V. Classification of diabetic angioneuropathy of the lower extremities. //Surgery. -2001. -№2. -c.43-45.
9. Afanasyev A.N. Interrelation of POL-AOH processes and immunity in patients with diabetic suppurative osteoarthropathy // First Belarusian International Congress of Surgeons. -Vitebsk. -1996.-C.363-365.
10. Akhmedov R.M., Safoev B.B., Khamdamov B.Z. Possibilities and prospects of application of the improved method of lower limb amputation in diabetic foot syndrome with critical ischaemia. -Surgery of Uzbekistan. -2008. -№2. -C. 5-8.
11. Bababekov A.R. Improvement of methods of treatment of diabetic gangrene of lower limbs (according to the data of distant results). Abstract of dissertation. Candidate of medical sciences - Tashkent, 2002, p 23.
12. Babadjanov B.D., Islamov M.S., Zhanabaev B.B. et al. Application of long-term intra-arterial catheter therapy in the treatment of purulent necrotic lesions of the foot in patients with diabetes mellitus. //Pathology. -2000. -№4. -C.52-53.
13. Babadjanov B.R., Yakubov F.R., Sabirova M.U. Modern physical methods of action in complex treatment of patients with diabetes mellitus. -Surgery of Uzbekistan. -2006. -№2. -C. 75-76.

14. Baranov V.L., Rusakov V.F. Diabetic foot syndrome. Textbook. -Saint-Petersburg. -2000. -c. 47.
15. Belitsky A.G. Complex treatment of soft tissue diseases in patients with diabetes mellitus with correction of immunological disorders. Author's thesis, Candidate of Medical Sciences -Moscow. -1986. -24c.
16. Belov V.V., Bordunovsky V.N., Grekova N.M. et al. Effect of short-term immunosuppression on skin grafts engraftment in diabetic foot syndrome. //Vestn. Khir. -2008. - №5. -str. 32-36.
17. Belopolsky AA, Gertsen AV, Vasina TA Quantum methods in the treatment of patients with diabetic angiopathy. //First Belarusian International Congress of Surgeons. -Vitebsk. -1996. -C.369-370.
18. Belyaev A.N., Rygin E.A., Zakhvatov A.N. et al. Systemic and regional antioxidant therapy in complicated forms of diabetic foot. Surgery, 2007, No. 11, pp. 46-51.
19. Bensman V.M., Galenko-Yaroshevsky , Mehta S.K., Triandafilov K.V. Prevention of limb amputations in patients with a complication of the "diabetic foot." //Surgery. -1999. -№10. -c.49-52.
20. Bregovsky V.B., Zaitsev A.A., Zalevskaya A.G., et al. Lesion of the lower extremities in diabetes mellitus. S-Pb.: "Dilya", 2004; p. 234
21. Bregovsky V.B., Tsvetkova T.L., Lebedev V.V.. Clinical and biomechanical characteristics of diabetic patients with Charcot arthropathy. // "Surgery 2000." -Moscow. -2000. -c.491-492.
22. Briskin B.S., Tartakovsky E.A., Gvozdev N.A. et al. Treatment of complications "diabetic foot." //Surgery. -1999. -№10. -c.53-57.
23. Briskin B.S., Sakunova T.I., Proshin A.V. et al. The use of pectin in the local treatment of the wound process in patients with diabetes mellitus. // "Surgery 2000. -Moscow. -2000. -c.494-495.
24. Vartanyan K.F. Clinical and diagnostic aspects of osteopathy in diabetes mellitus //Russian Medical News. -2003. -№3. -C.39-46.
25. Volynskaya S.V. Diagnostic significance of ultrasound Doppler in the detection of lesions of the main arteries in diabetes mellitus. //3rd Congress of the Russian Association of specialists of ultrasound diagnostics in medicine. -Moscow. -1999. -c.41.
26. Vyrenkov Y.E., Teberdiev Y.B. Endolymphatic antibiotic therapy in patients with diabetes mellitus. // "Surgery 2000". -Moscow. -2000. -p.504
27.Gavrilenko V.G.,Stadnikov A.A., Yesipov V.K., Mitkin A.F. Application of oxytocin in complex treatment at purulent necrotic lesions of feet in patients with diabetes mellitus. //Vestn. hir. -2000. -№3. -c.59-62.

28. Gazetov B.M., Kalinin A.P. Surgical diseases in patients with diabetes mellitus. -M. Medicine. -1991. -256 c.
29. Gazin I.K. Informativeness of markers in assessing the severity of endotoxicosis in purulent-necrotic lesions of the lower extremities in patients with diabetes mellitus. //Clinical Laboratory Diagnostics. -2008. -№12. - pp. 17-19.
30. Gazin I.K. Pathophysiological aspects of endotoxicosis in patients with diabetes mellitus complicated by purulent infection of the foot and its correction at traditional treatment and treatment with the use of of ozonated physiological solution. //Pathological physiology and experimental therapy. -2008. -№4. -str. 23-25.
31. Gazin I.K. Intoxication criteria in assessing the severity of endotoxemia, the effectiveness of ozone therapy and conventional treatment in patients with diabetes mellitus complicated by purulent-necrotic lesions of the lower extremities. //Clinical Laboratory Diagnostics. -2008. -№6. - pp. 21-24.
32. Golbraikh V.A., Starkov S.V. Prospects of treatment of patients with diabetic foot syndrome. Vestn. Khir. 2003, No. 4, pp. 113-115.
33. Gostishev V.K., Khokhlov A.M., Afanasiev A.N., Kuleshov E.B.. Complex diagnosis and treatment of diabetic osteoarthropathies //First Belarusian International Congress of Surgeons. -Vitebsk. -1996. -C.379- 380.
34. Glyantsev S.P. Dressings with proteolytic enzymes in the treatment of purulent wounds. //Surgery. -1998. -№12. -c.32-37.
35. Grekova N.M., Lebedeva Y.V., Bordunovsky V.N. Method of improving the results of local operations for purulent-necrotic diseases of the foot in diabetes mellitus. Vestn. Khir. 2003, No. 5, pp. 78-81.
36. Grishin I.N., Kholodova E.A., Chur N.N. Surgical treatment of patients with diabetic foot. // News of Surgery. -1996. -N1. -C.3-7.
37. Gurieva I.V., Kuzina I.V., Voronin A.V. et al. Features of diagnosis and treatment of diabetic foot lesions. //Surgery. -1999. -№10. -c. 39.
38. Gurieva I.V., Kuzina I.V., Voronin A.V. et al. Diabetic foot syndrome. Method. Recommendations. -Moscow. -2000. -c.40.
39. Dadaev Sh.A., Dalimov Sh.S., Ashurmetov A.M., Saidazimov A. et al. Open method of treatment of purulent-necrotic wounds of lower limbs in patients with diabetes mellitus. //Conference of surgeons, endocrinologists, resuscitators. -Tashkent. -1996. -C.25-28.
40. Dedov I.I., Shestakova M.V. Diabetes mellitus. Moscow: Universum Publishing, 2003.
41. Dedov I.I., Udovichenko O.V., Galstyan G.R. Diabetic foot. Moscow:

Practical Medicine, 2005; 175.
42. Dedov I.I., Rozhinskaya L.Y., Belaya J.E. Role and place of bisphosphonates in the prevention and treatment of osteoporosis // Osteoporosis and Osteopathies. -2005.
№1. -C.20-27.
43. Dedov I.I., Shestakova M.V. Maksimova M.A Federal target programme. "Diabetes Mellitus". M.: Ministry of Health of the Russian Federation, Federal Diabetology Centre of the Russian Federation, ENC RAMS, 2002.
44. Jamalov S.I. Transplantation of pancreatic islet cells in the complex treatment of "diabetic foot" syndrome. Dissertation. Candidate of medical sciences - Tashkent. -1999. -133str.
45. Dzhumabaev S.U., Musashayhov H.T., Aleksandrov N.G. et al. Justification and application of regional lymphatic therapy in purulent-necrotic lesions of the foot in patients with diabetes mellitus. //Republican conference with international participation. -Andijan. - 1995.
46. Dibirov M.D., Gadzhimuratov R.U., Evseev Y.N., Novoseltsev O.S. Treatment of purulent-necrotic complications in diabetic macroangiopathy. //Surgery. -2001. -№3. -c.29-33.
47. Dreval A.V., Savitskaya K.I., Bakharev I.V. et al. Experience of using the drug "Curiosin" in the treatment of flaccid granulating ulcers in diabetic foot syndrome. // "Surgery 2000". -Moscow. -2000. -c.514-515.
48. Duboshina T.B., Yaylakhanyan K.S. Optimisation of surgical treatment of patients with complicated forms of diabetic foot. //Vestn. Khir. - 2008. -№2. -str. 98-100.
49. Efimov A.S. Diabetic angiopathy. //M. Medicine. -1989. -288 c.
50.Zhanabaev B.B. Improvement of the local methods of surgical treatment at purulent-necrotic lesions of diabetic foot. Abstract of dissertation. Candidate of medical sciences - Tashkent, 1997. C.15.
51. Zemlyanoy A.B. Purulent-necrotic forms of diabetic foot syndrome. Pathogenesis, diagnostics, clinic, treatment: clinical and laboratory research. Avtoref. dissertation. doctor of medical sciences, M. -2003. -45 pp.
52. Zemlyanoy A.B., Paltsyn A.A., Svetukhin A.M. et al. Rationale and variants of tactics of complex surgical treatment of purulent-necrotic forms of "diabetic foot". //Surgery. -1999. -№10. - c.44-48.
53. Ibragimov T.K. True prevalence of diabetes mellitus among the population of Uzbekistan and measures of its prevention. //II International Congress of Diabetologists of Central Asia. Theses of reports. -Tashkent. - 1996. -C.12.
54. Ivanov V.V., Seliverstov D.V., Sokolov A.V., Gausman B.Ya. Comparative

evaluation of the adaptation effect of laser therapy, extracorporeal ultraviolet blood irradiation, hyperbaric oxygenation and plasmapheresis in patients with diabetic foot. // "Surgery 2000". -Moscow. -2000. -c.520-521.
55. Izmailov G.A., Tereshchenko V.Y., Izmailov S.G. et al. Complex treatment of purulent-necrotic lesions of soft tissues and gangrene of the lower extremities in patients with diabetes mellitus. //Surgery. -1998. -
№2. -c.39-42.
56. Izmailov S.G., Izmailov G.A., Averyanov M.Yu. et al. Drug for local treatment of diabetic ulcers. // "Surgery 2000". -Moscow. -2000.
-c.524-525.
57. Isaev M.U., Abdul G., Chirko V.Yu. et al. Proteolytic enzyme of plant nature - papain. -T. "Uzbekistan." -2000. -C.127.
58. Islamov B.F. Treatment of insulin-dependent diabetes mellitus by transplantation of pancreatic islet cells. Author's thesis, Doctor of medical sciences - Tashkent. -1998. -c.36.
59. Islamov M.S. Pathogenetic substantiation and development of original sparing approaches to treatment of diabetic gangrene of lower limbs. Dissertation of Doctor of Medical Science - Tashkent. -2002. -c. 253.
60. Ismailov S.I., Nugmanova L.B., Babakhanov B.H., Rakhimzhanov O.N. Normative indicators of phosphorus-calcium metabolism and bone mineral saturation in residents of Uzbekistan. //Vestn. of General Practitioner. 1998. №3. C.11-13.
61. Ismailov S.I., Shamansurova Z.M., Kamalov T.T. et al. Diabetic foot syndrome. Tashkent, 2005, pp. 63.
62. Kazimirov L.I. Komarov N.V. Gorbunov S.N. Effect of ultraviolet irradiation of blood on the body. //Surgery. -1987. -№1. -c.103-108.
63. Kamalov T.T. Effectiveness of long-term intra-arterial catheter therapy in the treatment of purulent-necrotic lesions of the foot at diabetes mellitus. Author's thesis of candidate of medical sciences. -Tashkent. -1997. -c.17.
64. Karimov Sh.I., Babadjanov B.D., Ismailov A.S. et al. A new method of foot resection in diabetic gangrene of lower limbs.
//Republican conference with international participation. -Andijan. - 1995.
65. Karimov Sh.I., Babadjanov B.D., Islamov M.S. et al. Long-term results of long-term intra-arterial catheter therapy in the treatment of diabetic gangrene of the lower extremities. //Surgery of Uzbekistan. -2001. -№2. -c.24-27.
66. Karimov Sh.I., Babadjanov B.D., Islamov M.S. Diabetic gangrene of lower limbs. - T.: Izd. "Shark". 2003. -240c.
67. Kistauri A.G. Echoosteometric evaluation of the effectiveness of

osteoporosis therapy in patients with diabetes mellitus. //I-Congress of the Russian Association of Ultrasound Diagnostics Specialists in Medicine. - Moscow. -1991. -C. 133.
68. Kosinets A.N., Bulavkin V.P., Lopoukhov G.D., Zuahara Bassam et al. Differentiated approach to the diagnosis of clinical variants "Diabetic Foot"//First Belarusian International Congress of Surgeons.-Vitebsk. -1996.-C.412-413.
69. Krivikhin V.T., Osokin V.V., Pavlenko V.V. et al. Revascularising osteotrepanation in patients with diabetic foot. // "Surgery 2000". - Moscow. -2000. -c.530-532.
70. Krotov N.F., Akhtaev A.R., Kamalov T.T. et al. Effect of long-term intra-arterial catheter therapy on angioarchitectonics in diabetic gangrene of the lower extremities. //Republican conference with international participation. -Andijan. -1995.
71. Kohan E.P. Batranov V.A. Mitroshin G.E. Kohan V.E. Lumbar sympathectomy in patients with obliterating atherosclerosis of the arteries of the lower extremities with diabetes mellitus. //Klin.hir. -1990. -№7. -C.69- 70.
72. Kuleshov E.V. Principles of treatment of surgical diseases in elderly and senile persons suffering from diabetes mellitus. //Surgery. -2001.- №7. -c.34-39.
73. Kuliev R.A., Babaev R.F., Fattaev M.D., Alekperova N.V. Effect of physical factors of treatment on lipid peroxidation in surgical infection in patients with diabetes // Surgery. -1991. -N7. -C.20-23.
74. Leontieva N.V., Belotserkovsky M.V., Rostova N.S. et al. Photohemocorrection in complex treatment of patients with obliterative atherosclerosis of lower limb arteries. //Vestn. hir. -2000. -№6. - c.57-60.
75. Lipatov K.V., Sopromadze M.A., Emelyanov A.Y., Kanorsky I.D. Use of physical methods in the treatment of purulent wounds. //Surgery - 2001. -№10.-c.56-60.
76. Lokhvitsky SV, Darwin VV, Begezhanov BA, Morozov ES Comprehensive surgical treatment of patients with diabetic purulent osteoarthropathy of the lower extremities. // First Belarusian International Congress of Surgeons. - Vitebsk. -1996. -C.428-430.
77. Martov Y.B., Podolinsky S.G. Modern methods of prevention and treatment of diabetic angiopathy. // News of Surgery. -1996. -N1. -C.46- 54.
78. Markevich Yu.A., Boyko N.I., Pavlovsky M.P. Risk factors in the development of trophic ulcers in patients with diabetic foot syndrome. // "Surgery 2000". -Moscow. -2000. -c.546-547.

79. International agreement on diabetic foot. Compiled by the International Working Group on Diabetic Foot. M.: Bereg, 2000. 80.Mezhlumyan L.G., Kasymova T.D., Yuldashev P.H. Proteinases from milky of Carica papaya juice. //Chemistry of natural compounds. -2003. -№3. -C.171.
81. Mehmanov Sh. Application of ultraviolet-autoblood in the complex treatment of purulent-necrotic processes in patients with diabetes mellitus. Author's thesis. Candidate of medical sciences - Tashkent. -1992. -C.20.
82. Musashayhov H.T. Optimisation of complex treatment of purulent diseases in diabetes mellitus by using methods of efferent and lymphatic therapy. Author's thesis. D. M. Sc. -Tashkent. -2002. -c.34
83. Norchaev J.A., Azizkhanov A.T., Khusainov Y.U. Ultrasonic cavitation in the treatment of purulent wounds. I-Congress of young scientists-medics and doctors of Uzbekistan. Andijan 1991 p.101-102.
84. Norchaev J.A., Rakhmanov R.K., Sagatov M.M. Ultrasonic cavitation in the treatment of purulent wounds. Conference "Wounds and wound infection". Andijan, 1995.
85. Norchaev J.A., Rakhmanov R.K., Gaffarov N. Clinical approbation of a new enzyme preparation Kukumazim in the treatment of diabetic gangrene of the lower extremities. Conference "Wounds and wound infection". Andijan, 1995.
86. Norchaev J.A., Rakhmanov R.K., Sagatov M.M. Complex treatment of diabetic foot. 1st Congress of Belarusian Surgeons, Vitebsk, 1996 p.445-447.
87. Norchaev J.A., Rakhmanov R.K., Sagatov M.M. Intra-arterial injection of drugs in the treatment of diabetic gangrene. 1st Congress of Belarusian Surgeons, Vitebsk, 1996, p.447-448.
88. Norchaev J.A., Rakhmanov R.K., Sagatov M.M. USC of antiseptic solutions in the treatment of diabetic phlegmon of lower limbs. 1st Congress of Belarusian Surgeons, Vitebsk, 1996 p.448-449.
89. Norchaev J.A., Rakhmanov R.K., Gaffarov N. Treatment of diabetic gangrene of the lower extremities. I Congress of the Pirogov Association of Surgeons. Tashkent, 1996 p. 44-45
90. Norchaev J.A., Rakhmanov R.K., Sagatov M.M. Basic principles of treatment of diabetic gangrene of lower limbs. Conference "Surgical pathology on the background of diabetes mellitus" Tashkent, 1996 p.96-98.
91. Norchayev J.A., Rakhmanov R.K., Soatov M.M. New Enzymatic preparation Kukumazim in the treatment of pyoinflamattory diseases of soft tisseus. 13th national gastroenterology congress. Turkey, 1996.
92. Norchayev J.A., Rakhmanov R.K., Elmuratov Sh.M., Abdurakhmanov Kh. Regional infusion of pharmacology drugs in the suupurative disease of lower

extremities. International surgery congress.Tel-Aviv Israel. 1998.c.37-38.
93. Norchayev J.A., Rakhmanov R.K., Elmuratov Sh.M. Clinicals Trials of a new Kukumazim enzime suppurative surgery. International surgery congress.Tel-Aviv Israel. 1998. p.37-38.
94. Norchayev J.A., Rakhmanov R.K., Abdurakhmanov Kh., Yuldashev P.Kh. Local Enzime Therapy in purulent Surgery. Third international symposium on the chemistry of natural compounds. Bukhara, 1998. C.98.
95. Norchaev J.A., Rakhmanov R.K., Abdurakhmanov H.K., Yuldashev P.H. Study of microflora in patients with diabetic foot on the background of enzyme therapy with Kukumazim. Chemistry of Natural Compounds, Special Issue, 1998. p. p. 149-150. 149-150.
96. Norchaev J.A., Rakhmanov R.K., Abdurakhmanov H.K., Kasimova T.E. Influence of enzyme therapy with Kukumazim on indices of integral rheography in patients with diabetic foot. Chemistry of Natural Compounds, Special Issue, 1998. 150-151.
97. Norchaev J.A., Rakhmanov R.K., Abdurakhmanov H.K., Yuldashev P.H. New enzyme preparation Kukumazim in purulent-septic surgery. Chemistry of Natural Compounds, Special Issue, 1998. 153-154.
98. Norchaev J.A., Rakhmanov R.K., Abdurakhmanov H.K., Yuldashev P.H. Modern principles of diabetic gangrene treatment. Surgery of Uzbekistan, 1999, No. 2, pp. 72-75.
99. Norchaev J.A., Rakhmanov R.K., Abdurakhmanov H.K., Yuldashev P.H. Proteolytic enzymes in the treatment of purulent-necrotic diseases of soft tissues. Surgery of Uzbekistan, 2000, №4 p. 93-96. 93-96.
100. Norchaev J.A. Prevention and treatment of phantom pain syndrome after high amputations of the n/k in patients with diabetes mellitus. Neurology, 2001, No.1 p.49-50.
101. Norchaev J.A. Diabetic neuropathy. Neurology, 2001, No.3, pp.49-52.
102.Norchaev ZH.A., Rakhmanov R.K., Abdurakhmanov H.K., Sagatov M.M. Intra-arterial injection medicines preparations treatment of diabetic foot. Surgery of Uzbekistan 2001,No.2 p.93-95.
103. Norchaev J.A., Rakhmanov R.K., Abdurakhmanov H.K. Treatment of wet diabetic gangrene of the lower extremities. 3rd Congress of the Association of CIS surgeons named after Pirogov, Moscow, 2001. Pirogov, Moscow, 2001, p.187.
104. Norchaev J.A., Rakhmanov R.K., Abdurakhmanov H.K. Application of Kukumazim in purulent surgery. 3rd Congress of the Association of CIS surgeons named after Pirogov, Moscow, 2001. Pirogov, Moscow, 2001, p.188-

189.
105. Norchaev J.A., Rakhmanov R.K., Kayumov T.H., Abdurakhmanov H.K. Local treatment of purulent wounds. Surgery of Uzbekistan No.2 2002 P. 84-85.
106. Norchaev J.A., Rakhmanov R.K., Kayumov T.H. Treatment of purulent complications after high thigh amputations in patients with diabetes mellitus. Bulletin of Surgery named after I.I.Grekov, 2002. I.I.Grekov, 2002, No.2 p.90-91.
107. Norchaev J.A., Rakhmanov R.K., Kayumov T.H. Intra-arterial injection of drugs in the treatment of purulent-necrotic diseases of the lower limbs. Surgery of Uzbekistan No.4, 2002, pp.75-77.
108. Norchaev J.A., Rakhmanov R.K., Ismailov S.N., Kayumov T.H., Kamalovv T.T. Intra-arterial injection of drugs in the treatment of thrombo-littering and purulent-necrotic diseases of the lower extremities. Methodical recommendations, Tashkent, 2003. p.30.
109. Norchaev J.A., Rakhmanov R.K., Kayumov T.H. Diabetic foot syndrome. Methodological recommendations, Tashkent, 2003. p.32.
110. Norchaev J.A., Rakhmanov R.K., Kayumov T.H. Surgical treatment of diabetic foot syndrome. Surgery of Uzbekistan, 2003, No.4. C.76-79.
111. Norchaev J.A. New direction of surgical treatment of diabetic suppurative osteoarthropathy. Actual issues of reconstructive surgery, Tashkent, 2004, 117 pp.
112. Norchaev J.A. Clinical study of the action of the enzyme preparation cucumazyme in the treatment of trophic ulcers of the lower limbs in patients with diabetes mellitus. Reports of the Academy of Sciences Ruz, 2004, No.5, pp.67-70.
113. Norchaev J.A. Analgesia in small amputations of the foot in patients with diabetes mellitus. Problems of Biology and Medicine, 2004, No. 3, pp. 77-78.
114. Norchaev J.A. Diagnosis, classification and treatment of diabetic osteoarthropathy. "Osteoinductive approaches in traumatology and orthopaedics" Tashkent. 2005г. C.256-259.
115. Norchaev J.A. Maloinvasive urgent diagnostic measures in purulent-necrotic lesions of the foot in patients with diabetes mellitus. Actual problems of organisation of emergency medical aid. Tashkent, 2005.
116. Norchaev J.A. Echoosteometric and chemical studies of foot bones in diabetic foot syndrome. Surgery of Uzbekistan, 2005, No. 3, pp. 74-76.
117. Norchaev J.A. Complex treatment of ischaemic form of purulent necrotic lesions of lower limbs in patients with diabetes mellitus taking into account micro and macroangiopathy. "Actual issues of specialised surgery", Tashkent,

2007, P.167.
118. Norchaev J.A., Ataliev A.E., Shotemirov V.Kh. Purulent complications after thigh amputation in patients with diabetes mellitus. "Issues of nosocomial infection in emergency medicine". Samarkand, 2008.
119. Norchaev J.A. Clinical and radiological, chemical and echosteometric characteristics of diabetic osteoarthropathy. Problems of Biology and Medicine, 2008, No. 2-1, pp. 61-63.
120. Norchaev ZH.A.. Determination degree severity purulent-necrotic process on the foot in diabetes mellitus. Klinichna Khirurgiya, 2009, No. 9, pp. 36-37.
121.Norchaev ZH.A.Algorithm therapeutic-diagnostic measures in diabetic foot syndrome. Klinichna Khirurgiya, 2009, No. 10, pp. 33-35.
122. Norchaev J.A. Estimation of severity of diabetic foot syndrome. Problems of Biology and Medicine, 2010, No. 1, pp. 94-96.
123. Norchaev J.A., Babadjanov B.D. Clinical and radiological characteristics of bone and joint changes in diabetic foot syndrome. Materials of the 2nd Congress of Traumatologists of Moscow, Moscow, 2014, p.202-203. 124.Norchaev J.A., Babadjanov B.D. Diagnosis, classification and treatment of diabetic osteoarthropathy. Materials of the 2nd Congress of Traumatologists of Moscow, Moscow, 2014, p.200-201.
125. Norchaev J.A., Babadjanov B.D. Treatment of trophic ulcers of the lower extremities in patients with diabetes mellitus. Medical Journal of Uzbekistan, 2014, No.4, pp.11-13.
126. Norchaev J.A. Pathogenesis of diabetic osteoarthropathy. Medical Journal of Uzbekistan, 2014, No.4, P.24-26.
127. Norchaev J.A. Clinical manifestations of various forms of diabetic foot syndrome. Materials of the scientific and practical conference "Actual problems of traumatology and orthopaedics" Samarkand, 2014, pp.335-336.
128. Norchaev J.A., Babadjanov B.D. Methods of foot unloading in diabetic osteoarthropathy. Materials of scientific and practical conference "Actual problems of traumatology and orthopaedics" Samarkand, 2014, p.264-265.
129. Norchaev J.A. Standardisation of therapeutic and diagnostic measures in diabetic foot syndrome. "Actual problems of traumatology and orthopaedics" Samarkand, 2014, pp.342-344.
130. Norchaev J.A. Treatment of diabetic osteoarthropathy. Medical Journal of Uzbekistan, 2015, No.2 P.27-30.
131. Norchaev J.A. Chemical analysis of bones in diabetic foot syndrome. "Ilizarov Readings", Russia, Kurgan, 2015.

132. Norchaev J.A. Treatment of trophic ulcers of the lower extremities in patients with diabetes mellitus. "Ilizarov Readings", Russia, Kurgan, 2015.
133. Norchaev ZH.A.Diabetic neuroosteoarthropathy. "Ilizarov Readings", Russia, Kurgan, 2015.
134. NorchaevZH.A. Ibn Sino o treatment diabetic osteoarthropathy. Legacy of Ibn Sina in the development of modern medicine, Termez, 2015.
135. Norchaev J.A. Features of blood flow in the lower limbs in diabetic osteoarthropathy. TMA Bulletin, 2019, Special Issue, pp. 74.
136. Norchaev J.A. Clinical and neurological features of the pathogenesis of diabetic neuroosteoarthropathy. Neurology, 2020, No. 1, pp. 42-44.
137. Norchayev J.A. Using vegetable proteolytic enzyme cucumazimum in treatment trophic ulcer of the lower limbs in patients with sugar diabetes. XIX scientific and practical conference with international participation "Metabolism in adaptation and damage - days of clinical and laboratory diagnostics on Don", Rostov, Russia, 2020.
138. Norchaev J.A. Complex treatment of diabetic neuroosteoarthropathy. Neurology, 2020, No. 4, pp.
139. Norchaev J.A. Addition to the classification of diabetic foot syndrome.Journal of Medicine and Innovations, 2021, No.2, pp. 50-53.
140. Norchaev J.A. Immunomorphological characteristics of the course of diabetic foot syndrome. Journal of Medicine and Innovations, 2021, No. 2, pp. 98-102.
141. Norchaev J.A. Morphological characteristics of the course of diabetic foot syndrome. Conference dedicated to the 95th anniversary of the birth of Academician Zufarov K. Tashkent, 2021.
142. Norchaev J.A. Morphological characteristics of the course of diabetic foot syndrome. Journal "New Day in Medicine", 2022, No. 4(42), pp. 189-191.
143. Norchaev J.A. Natural remedies in the treatment of diabetic neuroosteoarthropathy. XXI Interregional Scientific and Practical Conference "Metabolism in Adaptation and Damage - Days of Clinical Laboratory Diagnostics on Don" Rostov, Russia.
144. Norchaev J.A., Khamdamov S.I., Rakhmonov O.R. Predicting the course of diabetic foot syndrome. THE JOURNAL 2022, NO.2. Pages 245- 249.
145. Norchaev J.A, Khamdamov Sh.I. Predicting the course of diabetic foot syndrome. International Conference on Developments in Education Hosted from Amsterdam, Netherlands 2022 190-194.
146. Norchaev J.A. Diabetic osteoarthropathy. Monograph. LAP Lambert Academic Publishing, 2022. 70 pp.

147. Norchaev J.A. Natural remedies in the treatment of diabetic neuroosteoarthropathy. Journal of Innovation, Creativity and Art Special Issue. 2023, 319-323.

148. Pavlov Yu.I. Analysis of the main causes of low efficiency of care in purulent-necrotic complications of diabetic foot syndrome. //Vestn. Khir. -2007. -№5. -str. 28-32.

149. Pavlov Y.I., Kholopov A.A., Sidorenko I.K. Standardisation is effective in the treatment of purulent-necrotic forms of diabetic foot. //International Electronic Journal of Nursing. -2002.

150. Pavlova M.G., T.V. Gusov, N.V. Lavrishcheva. Diabetic foot syndrome. //Trudny Patient. -2006, -№1. -C. 27-31.

151. Piksin I.N., Atyasov N.I., Kiseleva R.E. et al. Ultraviolet irradiation of blood in surgery. //Surgery. -1990. -№11. -c.100-102.

152. Pupyshev M.L. Surgical treatment of non-destructive and destructive lesions of the feet in patients with diabetes mellitus. // Abstract of the dissertation... Dr.m.n. -Novosibirsk. -2001. -c.27.

153. Rakhimov M.R. Pharmacological study of domestic proteolytic enzyme papain. // Author's thesis D. M. Sc. - Tashkent. - 2001. -c.28.

154. Rakhimova G.N. Early stages of diabetes mellitus types 1 and 2 (features of pathogenesis, diagnosis, treatment and prevention). //Author abstract of dissertation... Doctor of medical sciences, -Tashkent. -2002. -c.39.

155. Rogachev V.A. Intra-arterial insulin therapy in the complex treatment of purulent-necrotic forms of diabetic foot. // "Surgery 2000". -Moscow. -2000. -c.577-579.

156. Svetukhin A .M., Zemlyanoy A .B. Diabetic foot syndrome. //Materials of the V Russian Scientific Forum "Surgery - 2004". M. 2004. -str. 175-178.

157. Svetukhin A.M., Zemlyanoy A.B., Koltunov V.A. Long-term results of treatment of patients with purulent-necrotic forms of diabetic foot syndrome. //Surgery. -2008. -№7. -str. 8-10.

158. Diabetic foot syndrome. Report of the Endocrinological Research Centre of the Russian Academy of Medical Sciences. -2007. C.55.

159. Slesarenko S.S., Frankfurt L.A., Eremenko S.M. Application of ultrasound cavitation and specific application therapy in the complex treatment of purulent wounds. //Surgery. -1998. -№8. -c.25-26.

160. Udovichenko O . V., Antsiferov M . B. Diabetic osteoarthropathy. //The Treating Physician. -2002. -№5. -C. 30-34.

161. Udovichenko O.V., Galstyan G.R. Immobilising unloading dressing (total contact cast) in the treatment of trophic ulcers in patients with diabetes // Diabetes Mellitus. 2003. № 3. C. 29-34.
162. Ulyanova I.N., Macherets E.A., Tokmakova A.Yu. Biochemical markers of bone metabolism in differential diagnostics of haematogenous osteomyelitis and acute stage of diabetic osteoarthropathy. Vestn. Khir. 2003, No. 4, pp. 34-37.
163. Chur N.N., Grishin I.N., Kazlovskiy A.A., Kokoshko Y.I. Etiology, pathogenesis, classification and surgical treatment of diabetic foot syndrome. //Surgery. 2003. №4. C.42-46.
164. Shaposhnikov V.I., Zorik V.V.. Combined treatment of purulent-necrotic lesions of the lower limbs in diabetes mellitus.
//Surgery. -2001. -№2. -c.46-49.
165. Shaposhnikov Y.G., Rudakov B.Y., Berchenko G.N. et al. Complex treatment of purulent wounds using UV-irradiation of blood. //Surgery. - 1988. - №4. -c.17-21.
166. Shor N.A. Surgical tactics in diabetic angiopathy of the lower extremities with purulent-necrotic lesions. //Surgery. -2001. -№6. - c.29-33.
167. Shulutko A.M., Antropova N.V., Kruger Yu.A. NO therapy in patients with diabetes mellitus complicated by purulent-necrotic lesions of the lower extremities. //Surgery. - 2004. - №12. - pp. 43-46.
168. Acton KJ, Shields R, Rith-Najarian S, Tolbert B, Kelly J, Moore K, Valdez L, Skipper B, Gohdes D. Applying the diabetes quality improvement project indicators in the Indian Health Service primary care setting. : Diabetes Care 2001 Jan;24(1):22- 26.
169. Ali SM, Basit A, Sheikh T, Mumtaz S, Hydrie MZ. Diabetic foot ulcer-a prospective study. J Pak Med Assoc 2001 Feb;51(2):78-81.
170. American Diabetes Association. Standards of medical care in diabetes-2007. Diabetes Care. 2007; 30(Suppl.1):S4-S41.
171. American Diabetes Association. Standards of medical care in diabetes - 2008. Diabetes Care. 2008;31:S12-S54.
172. American Diabetes Association (ADA). Standards of medical care in diabetes.
IV. Prevention/delay of type 2 diabetes. Diabetes Care. 2007;30:S7-S8.
173. Andel M. [Diabetology at the threshold of the 21st century]. : Vnitr Lek 2001 May;47(5):277-280.
174. Apelqvist J. What is the most effective way to reduce incidence of amputation in the diabetic foot? // Diabetes metab. Rev. -2000. -Vol. 16. №1/ -P. 75-83.

175. Bakker DJ. Hyperbaric oxygen therapy and the diabetic foot. Diabetes Metab Res Rev 2000 Sep-Oct;16 Suppl 1:S55-58.
176. Bachmann MO, Eachus J, Hopper CD, et al. Socio-economic inequalities in diabetes complications, control, attitudes and health service use: a cross-sectional study. Diabet Med. 2003 Nov;20(11):921-9.
177. Barnett AH. A review of basal insulins. Diabet Med. 2003 Nov;20(11):873-85.
178. Benotmane A, Mohammedi F, Ayad F, Kadi K, Medjbeur S, Azzouz A. Management of diabetic foot lesions in hospital: costs and benefits. : Diabetes Metab 2001 Dec;27(6):688-694.
179. Calle-Pascual AL, Duran A, Diaz A, et al. Comparison of peripheral arterial reconstruction in diabetic and non-diabetic patients: a prospective clinic-based study. : Diabetes Res Clin Pract 2001 Aug;53(2):129-36.
180. Campbell LV, Graham AR, Kidd RM, et al. The lower limb in people with diabetes. Position statement of the Australian Diabetes Society. : Med J Aust 2000 Oct 2;173(7):369-372.
181. Caravaggi C, Faglia E, De Giglio R, et al. Effectiveness and safety of a nonremovable fibreglass off-bearing cast versus a therapeutic shoe in the treatment of Neuropathic foot ulcers: a randomised study. Diabetes Care 2000 Dec;23(12):1746- 1751.
182. Davies S, Gibby O, Phillips C, et al. The health status of diabetic patients receiving orthotic therapy. : Qual Life Res 2000 Mar;9(2):233-240.
183. Deery HG, Sangeorzan JA. Saving the diabetic foot with special reference to the patient with chronic renal failure. Infect Dis Clin North Am 2001 Sep;15(3):953-81.
184. Elftman NW. Orthotic management of the neuropathic limb. Phys Med Rehabil Clin N Am 2000 Aug;11(3):509-551.
185. Embil JM, Nagai MK. Becaplermin: recombinant platelet derived growth factor, a new treatment for healing diabetic foot ulcers. Expert Opin Biol Ther 2002 Feb;2(2):211-218.
186. Frykberg RG, Bailey LF, et al. Offloading properties of a rocker insole. A preliminary study. J Am Podiatr Med Assoc 2002 Jan;92(1):48-53.
187. Gazis A, Pound N, Macfarlane R, et al. Mortality in patients with diabetic neuropathic osteoarthropathy (Charcot foot). Diabet Med. 2004 Nov;21(11):1243-6.
188. Gonzalez ER, Oley MA. The management of lower-extremity diabetic ulcers. Manag Care Interface 2000 Nov;13(11):80-87.
189. Harrison AJ, Hillard PJ. A moment-based technique for the automatic

spatial alignment of plantar pressure data. Proc Inst Mech Eng [H] 2000;214(3):257-264.
190. Hartemann-Heurtier A, Marty L, Ha Van G, Grimaldi A. Role of antibiotic therapy in diabetic foot management. Diabetes Metab 2000 May;26(3):219-224.
191. Jirkovska A. [The diabetic foot syndrome--one of the most serious complications in diabetics]. : Vnitr Lek 2001 May;47(5):311-314.
192. Kreyden OP, Hafner J, Burg G, Nestle FO. Case report on therapy with granulocyte stimulating factor in diabetic foot. //Hautarzt 2001 Apr;52(4):327-330.
193. La Fontaine J, Reyzelman A, Rothenberg G, Husain K, Harkless LB. The role of revascularisation in transmetatarsal amputations. : J Am Podiatr Med Assoc 2001 Nov-Dec;91(10):533-535.
194. Murphy B.J.. ADA Recommendations for Foot Care in People with Diabetes March 13, 2005.
195. Plummer E.S., Albert S.G. Focused assesment of foot care in older adults. Journal of the American Geriatrics Society, 1996, 44(3), 310-313.
196. Sambrook P.N., Rodriguez J.P., Washnish R.D. et al. Alendronate in the prevention of osteoporosis: 7-year follow-up. //Osteoporosis International. - 2004. - Vol. 15 : 483-488.
197. Thomas SR, Perkins JM, Magee TR, Galland RB. Transmetatarsal amputation: an 8-year experience. Ann R Coll Surg Engl 2001 May;83(3):164-166.
198. Vayssairat M, Le Devehat C. [Diabetic angiopathy: the role of microvascular exploration in routine practice. Consequences of a new algorithm for care of the diabetic foot]. : J Mal Vasc 2001 Apr;26(2):126-129.
199. Wagner S, Reike H, Angelkort B. [Highly resistant pathogens in patients with diabetic foot syndrome with special reference to methicillin-resistant Staphylococcus aureus infections]. Dtsch Med Wochenschr 2001 Nov 30;126(48):1353-1356.

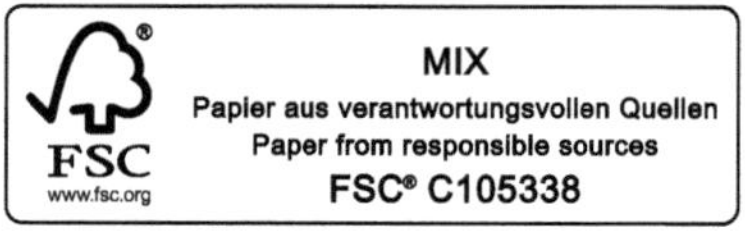

Printed by Books on Demand GmbH, Norderstedt / Germany